Positive Health
in
Tibetan Medicine

Indian Medical Science Series No. 13

Positive Health in Tibetan Medicine

based on
Sman–'tsho-ba'i mdo
(Vaidya–Jīva–sūtra)

Vaidya Bhagwan Dash
&
Ven. Doboom Tulku

SRI SATGURU PUBLICATIONS
A division of
INDIAN BOOK CENTRE
Delhi-India

Published by:
SRI SATGURU PUBLICATIONS
Indological & Oriental Publishers,
A Division of
INDIAN BOOKS CENTRE
40/5, Shakti Nagar,
Delhi-110007
INDIA

First Edition: 1991–Delhi
ISBN–81–7030–255-2

***Printed at*:**
D. K. Fine Art Press, Delhi.

PRINTED IN INDIA

Contents

*. Line nos. in parenthesis.

Foreword

It is a pleasure to observe the successful production of the Vaidya-Jīva-Sūtra from its extant Tibetan translation. Vaidya Bhagwan Dash now presents it in a form with Sanskrit words that are equivalent to the Tibetan terms, plus English translation, along with his own learned remarks.

Continuing the practice of Dash's numerous previous works, the names of the three '*dosha-s*,' namely, *vāyu, pitta,* and *kapha*, are left untranslated. The cogent reason is that the usual translations of the terms as are found in other books are based on the forms of the '*dosha*-s' after they depart from the body, whereas the terms mainly apply to the functions of the three in the body itself.

The high standard maintained in the present work reflects the many years devoted by Bhagwan Dash to Indo-Tibetan medicine in its various aspects, and on which he has published a number of very useful books. May the readers of this work profit from his admirable and intelligent industry.

Alex Wayman
Columbia University,
New York

Preface

In the Tangyur section of Tibetan scriptures several works on medicine (including Veterinary medicine) are incorporated. There are clear evidences in respect of most of these works that these were originally composed by Indian scholars in Sanskrit and subsequently translated into Tibetan language by Tibetan scholars, in some cases with the help of Indian scholars. Sanskrit originals of most of these works are no more extant. Since these works are in Tibetan language, Scientists, Physicians and well-meaning Research workers in other parts of the world are not able to study them and utilise them for the benefit of the suffering humanity.

The first work in this list, viz., *Sbyor-ba brgya-pa* or *Yoga Śataka*, with its translation in Sanskrit and English and notes has already been published by the Library of Tibetan Works and Archieves, Dharmashala, India in 1985. The seventh work in this list, viz., *Sman-bpyad Yan-lag brgyad-pa'i sñin po'i 'grel-pa las Sman-gyi Min-gi Rnam-grans* or *Vaidyaka Aṣṭāṅgahṛdayavṛttau Bheṣaja-Nāma-Paryāya* has also been published by Classics India Publications, New Delhi in 1986. The present work is placed second in the above mentioned list of works in the Tanjur scriptures and its Sanskrit or English translation is not yet attempted. Since this is an important work dealing with measures for the preservation and promotion of Positive health (which is a new concept in modern medicine) and prevention of diseases, we attempted to bring out its edition with English translation and notes in English.

Several editions (versions) of the Tanjur scriptures are available now. For collating and editing this text, we have used Derge, Narthang and Peking editions and given the variant readings in the foot-notes marked in parenthesis as (D), (N), and (P) respectively. In addition, we were fortunate to get an edition of this work in type print which was edited and published by Prof. J. Cai of the Academy of Traditional Chinese Medicine, Beijing in 1988. Even if Prof. Cai seems to have followed Derge edition, several important variant readings are available in this work which are incorporated in foot-notes with the mark (J).

We very much desired to give the Tibetan text in the original Tibetan script. But, because of non-availability of Tibetan types we had to Romanise them, and in this connection, we have followed the pattern of transliteration approved and adopted by the U.S. Library of Congress. Below each Tibetan term we have given the Sanskrit equivalent (without case endings) in Devanāgarī. After the English translation of the Tibetan text (and in some cases even before it), we have given brief notes in English to explain the topic.

This work is in verses except the initial invocation, introductory remarks and colophon. In the original Tibetan text, the verses are not numbered. We have numbered each line to facilitate reference and clubbed them together with main-headings or side-headings on the basis of topics discussed. It is perhaps necessary to mention here that in all these editions, there are errors inasmuch as several lines are not complete. Since this is a scriptural work and these errors might have crept into the text by calligraphers or cutters of wooden blocks, we have not taken the liberty to fill up the missing words. However, we have indicated such omissions and errors in our notes under the respective lines of the work.

The biggest hurdle in the translation of Tibetan works in general and medical works in particular is the difficulty in finding both Sanskrit and English equivalents of the Tibetan technical words. Therefore, at the end, we have furnished two indices incorporating such technical terms. In the first appendix, Tibetan terms (though Romanised), are arranged in Tibetan alphabetical order. In the second appendix, Sanskrit words (without case endings) are arranged according to the order of Devanāgarī.

This is only as humble attempt and we do not claim perfection. This can serve as a basic text which can be further improved and corrected by the future Research scholars.

Acknowledgements

Prof. Alex Wayman had kindly supplied us a zerox copy of the Derge edition of this work from his Library. He has also honoured us by writing a Foreword to this work. We are thankful to him for his guidance and encouragement. We are also thankful to Prof. J. Cai, whose edition of this work we have utilised.

New Delhi
15th March, 1991

BHAGWAN DASH
DOBOOM TULKU

INDO-ROMANIC EQUIVALENTS OF DEVANĀGARĪ AND TIBETAN LETTERS

Devanāgarī	*Tibetan*	*Indo-romanic*	*Devanāgarī*	*Tibetan*	*Indo-romanic*
अ	ཨ	a	च	ཙ་	ca
आ	(ཨཱ)	ā	छ	ཚ་	cha
इ	ཨི	i	ज	ཛ་	ja
ई	(ཨཱི)	ī	झ	(ཛྷ་)	jha
उ	ཨུ	u	ञ	ཉ་	ña
ऊ	(ཨཱུ)	ū	ट	(ཊ་)	ṭa
ऋ	-	ṛ	ठ	(ཋ་)	ṭha
ए	ཨེ	e	ड	(ཌ་)	ḍa
ऐ	(ཨཻ)	ai	ढ	(ཌྷ་)	ḍha
ओ	ཨོ	o	ण	(ཎ་)	ṇa
औ	(ཨཽ)	au	त	ཏ་	ta
ं	ཾ	ṁ	थ	ཐ་	tha
ः	ཿ	ḥ	द	ད་	da
क	ཀ་	ka	ध	(དྷ་)	dha
ख	ཁ་	kha	न	ན་	na
ग	ག་	ga	प	པ་	pa
घ	(གྷ་)	gha	फ	ཕ་	pha
ङ	ང་	ṅa	ब	བ་	ba

भ	(བྷ་)	bha	य	ཡ་	ya
म	མ་	ma	र	ར་	ra
(च़)	ཙ་	tsa	ल	ལ་	la
(छ़)	ཚ་	tsha	व	[ཝ་]	va
(ज़)	ཛ་	dza	श	ཤ་	śa
(व)	ཝ་	va	ष	(ཥ་)	ṣa
—	ཞ་	źa	स	ས་	sa
—	ཟ་	za	ह	ཧ་	ha
—	འ་	a'	[अ]	ཨ་	a

Introduction

In the recent past, modern medicine has made phenomenal progress in eradicating many infectious diseases and controlling several metabolic ailments, not withstanding the adverse toxic effects of some of the newly discovered remedies. But the basic problem of health lies not in curing diseases, and not even in their prevention because a person who is simply free from diseases is not to be treated as 'healthy' in the real sense of the term. In addition, he should be mentally and spiritually happy to lead a productive and socially useful as well as beneficial life till his inevitable death. He should be an asset with his accumulated experience and not a liability with his invalidating diseases for the society.

Health for All

The World Health Organisation has fixed its goal as "Health for All" by 2000 A.D.. It will be difficult to achieve this aim simply by increasing the number of medical colleges, hospitals and dispensaries and by producing more of doctors and paramedical staff. For this, it is essential to propagate the knowledge of and adopt the measures for the preservation and promotion of Positive Health and prevention of diseases.

Positive Health

The concept of "Positive Health" is in its infancy in modern medicine. On the other hand, in Tibetan medicine and in Ayurveda, this aspect, i.e. measures for positive health is more emphasised and elaborately described. Scientists all over the world are evincing keen interest in the Traditional medicines of different countries mainly to find a medicine or therapy for curing such diseases for which modern conventional medicines are not available or they produce adverse reactions as a result of which the patient suffers more because of these toxic reactions than the disease he was suffering from. But the concept of Positive Health dealing with measures to prevent the occurence of diseases and to make a person lead not only physically but mentally and spiritually happy life is relegated to a position of low priority. The main reason for this neglect is perhaps the absence of commercial value in the propagation of such measures. If a person falls ill, then several people including the scientists who discover new drugs, the industrialists who manufacture them, the physicians who prescribe them, and chains of distributors who supply these drugs through their several channels are benefitted. If measures to make a person lead a disease-free and happy life are propagated, then only the individual is benefited. In this materialistic world he is in a minority, and therefore, measures which are useful for him do not attract the elite attention. There is perhaps nothing to be surprised about it.

Distinctive Features of Tibetan Tradition

The religious, social and cultural traditions of Tibet are however, distint and different. They want an individual to be free from diseases, and mentally and spiritually happy. Therefore, they lay more emphasis upon positive health and prevention of disease for which several measures are prescribed and adopted in their day to day life.

Origin of Diseases

According to *Caraka* (*Caraka Saṃhitā* : *Vimāna* 3 : 24) sinful acts give rise to inauspiciousness. During the first age (*Satya Yuga*) people were enthusiastic, energetic, pure (free from sinful acts) and therefore powerful. They were endowed with the visions of the gods and divine saints. With the sense of duty, they performed religious rites. They were endowed with truthfulness, charity, self-control, observance of social rules, meditation and celibacy (*brahmacarya*). They were devoid of fear, attachment, envy, delusion, greed, anger, grief, mental afflictions, abnormal sleep, drowsiness, fatigue, exhaustion, laziness and tendency to collect and accumulate wealth. Because of these features, they were endowded with unlimited span of life. Because of the noble mind, qualities and actions of people, the earth, water, air, etc., were endowed with all good qualities as a result of which excellent tastes, potencies, *vipaka* (tastes which emerge after digestion) and specific actions were manifested in food grains. At the end of this age, some rich people got heaviness in their bodies because of over indulgence. They suffered from fatigue because of the heaviness in their body. Fatigue gave rise to laziness and this laziness made them to accumulate wealth. Accumulation of wealth lead to the attachment for such things and attachment resulted in greed.

During the second age (Treta Yu*ga*), greed gave rise to malice, malice gave rise to false statements and from these false statements arose passion, anger, vanity, dislike, cruelty, infliction of injuries, fear, sorrow, grief, worry, anxiety, etc. Because of these factors, the life span of human beings was reduced by a quarter. Similarly, there were diminutions in the attributes of earth, etc., and the attributes of drugs and food ingredients were less manifested.

Diseases Caused by Artificial Living

According to *Caraka* (*Caraka Saṃhitā* : *Cikitsā* : 1 : 4 : 3) persons living close to nature remained free from diseases. It is when they adopt various artificial modes of living that they succumbed to diseases and death. In the present day so called civilised world, civilisation has become synonymous with artificial living and behaviour. People who lead more and more of artificial way of living are considered more and more civilised. The pleasure that one gets in this artificial living is transitory and it inflicts more miseries in the long run. It is in the Nature lies the measures for healthy living. For maintaining Positive health, it is necessary to understand this nature properly. This includes the understanding of the changes the body undergoes during different seasons, different parts of the day and night, the effects of such changes on the body, mind and soul of the individual, and on the medicinal plants, ingredients of food and drinks.

Body and Universe Relationship

Body (micro-cosm) is a replica of the Universe (macro-cosm). Every aspect of the Universe is represented in the body of an individual of course in a subtle form. Therefore, any change in the environment affects the body, mind and spirit of the individual. On the other hand, every activity of the individual, through his body, mind and speech affects himself and his environment. A bad speech (spoken word), for example, will affect the individual and his environment. On the other hand, a good and auspicious speech will keep the individual healthy. Here comes the role of mantras and religious rites for the good health of people. The seed letters (*bīja akṣaras*) of a mantra, if repeatedly and devotedly recited in a prescribed manner, helps in the maintenence of various elements in the body in a state of equilibrium. This not only helps in the prevention and cure of diseases, but in addition, promotes positive health.

Body - Mind Relationship

According to Tibetan medicine and Ayurveda, both the body and the mind are closely interrelated inasmuch as the health, happiness and misery of one affects the other. This Psycho-somatic concept of disease and health is very important and basic to both these systems.

Psycho-Somatic Concept

The body of living beings is composed of *nad* or *ñes pa* or *doṣa* (which are three in number, viz., *rluṅ* or *vāyu*, *mkhris pa* or *pitta* and *bad kan* or *kapha*). *lus zuṅs* or *dhātu* (which includes seven categories of tissue elements) and *dri ma* or *mala* (which includes several types of waste products including *bśaṅ ba* or *purīṣa* or *stool*, *gci ba* or *mūtra* or urine and *rṅul* or *sveda* or sweat). If these are in a state of equilibrium in the body, then the person remains free from diseases. Out of the above mentioned three categories, the first one i.e. *ñes pa* or *doṣa* plays an important role in the causation and prevention of diseases. The three types of *ñes pa*, viz., *rluṅ* or *vāyu*, *mkhris* pa or *pitta* and *bad kan* or *kapha* are controlled by three mental factors, viz., '*dod chags* or *kāma* (passion), *że sdaṅ* or *krodha* (anger) and *gti mug* or *moha* (illusion) respectively. Thus, the mind and body are closely connected with each other. Psychic factors effectively control the physical factors and *vice versa*. The disease and for that matter health is explained on the basis of this psycho-somatic concept which is one of the unique features of Tibetan medicine and Ayurveda.

Holistic Concept

Different organs and tissue elements of the body may be structurally distinct and different. But their is functional unity among these various organs inasmuch as one particular organ can not remain healthy if others surrounding it are diceased. For the good health it is essential that all these organs should function harmoneously. If a particular organ is afflicted, while curing it, the health of other organs is also to be taken care of. The disease manifested in a particular part or organ of the body or faculty of mind can not be treated or prevented in isolation. Other parts of the body and mind are also to be looked into and corrected for the successful prevention and treatment of diseases. This holistic approach to the disease and health is one of the characteristic features of Tibetan medicine and Ayurveda.

Conglomeration of Science, Philosophy and Religion

In addition to several diet, drinks and regimens, Tibetan medicine and Ayurveda prescribe several conducts, manners and religious rites for maintaining health. One should not treat these factors as futile and narrow sectarianism or religious fanaticism. It is not necessary for a person to adopt Buddhism and for that matter Hinduism for keeping good health. The purpose of providing religious prescriptions simply indicates that a person, to keep himself healthy should sincerely follow the instructions of his own religious faith and without that it is well nay impossible for him to be healthy. Tibetan medicine and Ayurveda are the conglomerations of science, philosophy and religion.

Emphasis on Field than Seed

In Tibetan medicine and Ayurveda, more emphasis is laid upon 'field' than the 'seed'. A seed, if planted in fertile field and supplied with appropriate quantity of water, air and sun light can germinate and grow as a tree. But if it is placed over a barron land it will not be able to grow. The role of disease causing germs are well recognised in these systems. But germs (seeds) are considered to be secondary causes, the primary cause being the harmony of the various disease causing factors and tissue elements (field) inside the body. If *rluṅ* or *vāyu, mkhris pa* or *pitta* and *bad kan* or *kapha* are in a state of equilibrium, then the germ, howsoever virulant or powerful it may be, will not be able to produce a disease in the body. For the prevention and cure of diseases and for the maintenance of positive health, all the efforts in the form of drugs, diet, drinks including regimens and behaviour are directed towards maintaining this state of equilibrium.

Emphasis on Diet Drinks

For health, more emphasis is laid upon appropriate diet, drinks and regimens in comparison to drugs and therapies. It is stated, "If a person is on proper diet, etc., then there is no need for medicine and if a person is not on appropriate diet, then there is no need for medicine". In the former case, the diet will prevent and cure his diseases, and in the latter case, in spite of medicines and therapies the person will not be free from diseases. This is also one of the unique features of Tibetan medicine and Ayurveda.

Classification of Knowledge

According to the popular Tibetan tradition, all the religious and secular types of knowledge are grouped into ten categories. These are called *rig gnas* or *vidyā stāna*. Five of them form a group of major subjects as follows:

(1) *Bzo rig pa* or *Śilpa śāstra* (Technology)

(2) *Gso ba rig pa* or *Cikitsā śāstra* (Medicine)

(3) *Sgra'i rig pa* or *Śabda śāstra* (Grammar)

(4) *Tshad ma rig pa* or *Pramāṇa śāstra* (Logic)

(5) *Nań don rig pa* or *Dharma śāstra* (Religion)

The remaining five of them which form the group of minor subjects are as follows:

(1) *Sñan ṅag* or *Kāvya śāstra* (Poetics)

(2) *Sdeb sbyor* or *Chanda śāstra* (Metrics)

(3) *Mṅon brjod* (*Abhidhāna śāstra* (Lexicon)

(4) *Zlos gar* or *Nāṭya śāstra* (Dramatics)

(5) *Skar rtsis* or *Jyotiṣa śāstra* (Astrology)

The importance given to medicine lies in its inclusion in the group of major subjects and it is with this in view that several medical texts are incorporated in the Tanjur scriptures (a group of religious scriptures of Mahāyāna Buddhism), in addition to those prevalent in the noncanonical literature.

Medical Works in Religious Scriptures

Details of fourteen such medical works included in the Tanjur scriptures are as follows:

(1) Tibetan : *Sbyor-ba brgya-pa*
Sanskrit : *Yogaśataka.*
Author : Klu-sgrub-źabs (Nāgārjuna-pāda)
Translator : Jetakarṇa, Buddhaśrījñāna and Ñi-ma Rgyal-mtshan Bzaṅ-po.

(2) Tibetan : Sman-'tsho-ba'i mdo. (*Sman-'tsho'i mdo* or *Sman-bpyad 'tsho-ba'i mdo*)
Sanskrit : *Jīvasūtra* (*Vaidya Jīvasūtra*)
Author : Klu-sgrub Sñiṅ-po (Nāgārjuna-hṛdaya or Nāgārjuna-garbha).

(3) Tibetan : *Sman a-ba'i cho-ga.*
Sanskrit : *Avabheṣajakalpa*
Author : Klu-sgrub (Nāgārjuna).

(4) Tibetan : *Yan-lag brgyad-pa'i sñiṅ-po bsdus-pa*
Sanskrit : *Aṣṭaṅgahēdayasaṃhitā*
Author : Pha-khol (Vāgbhaṭa)
Translation : Jarandhara (Jālandhara) and Rin-chen bzaṅ-po.

(5) Tibetan : *Yan-lag brgyad-pa'i sñiṅ-po źes bya ba'i Sman-byad-kyi bsad-pa*
Sanskrit : *Aśṭāṅgahṛdaya-Vaidūryakabhāṣya*
Author : Pha-khol (Vāgbhaṭa)
Translation : Dharmaśrīvarman and Sakya blo-gros
Revisor : Rig-pa gźon-nu, Dbyig-gi Rin-chen.

(6) Tib. : *Yan-lag brgyad-pa'i sñiṅ-po'i rnam-par 'grel-pa tshig-gi don-gyi Zla-zer źes-bya-ba.*

San. : *Padārthacandrikā(prabhāṣā) nāma Aṣṭāṅgahṛdayvivṛti*

Auth. : Zla-ba-la dga'-ba (Candrnandana)

Tr. : Jalandhāra (Jalamdhara) and Rin-chen bzaṅ-po.

(7) Tib. : *Sman-*dpyad Yan-lag brgyad*-pa'i sñiṅ-po'i 'grel-pa las Sman-gyi miṅ gi rnam-graṅs.*

San. : *Vaidyaka Aṣṭāṅgahṛdaya-vṛttau Bheṣajanāmaparyāya*

Auth. : Zla-ba-la dga'-ba (Candranandana).

(8) Tib. : *Rta'i tshe'i rig'byed Sa-li-ho-tras bsdus-pa*

San. : *Ṣālihotrīya-Aśvāyurvedasaṃhitā*

Auth. : Ṣālihotra

Tr. : Ācārya Dharmaśrībhadra, Buddhaśrīśānti and Rin-chen bzaṅ-po.

(9) Tib. : *Sman-dpyad gces-pa grub-pa*

San. : *Vaidyaka-Siddhasāra.*

Auth. : Ñi-mas bsruṅs-pa (Ravigupta)

Tr. : Jīnamitra, Atirāgyavarman (Ādityavarman) and Candra.

10) Tib. : *'Phags-pa rtsa-ba'i mdzod-sman chen-po'i rim-pa*

San. : *Ārya-mūlakoṣa-Mahauṣadhāvalī*

Auth. : Klu-sgrub (Nāgārjuna)

Tr. : Chos-kyon bzaṅ-po.

(11) Tib. : *Tshe'i rig-byed mtha' dag-gi sñin-po bsdus-pa*

San. : *Āyurveda-sarvasva-sārasangraha*

Auth. : Tshans-sras Bshad-pa'i rdo rje (Brahmaputra-Hāsavajra)

Tr. : Khyim spans Sa-spyod, Nag-dban Phun-tshogs lhun-grub

Re. : Blo-bzan Chos-grags.

(12) Tib. : *'Phags-pa yul pha-ha'i sman-pa Da-na-da-sa'i Sman-bcos*

San. : *Āryadeśāpaha-bhiṣak Dānadāsa Bheṣajasaṃskāra.*

Auth. : Dānadāsa (Danadasa).

(13) Tib. : *Tshans-pa'i rig-byed rgya-mtsho'i Yan-lag 'dzin-pa Gyo-ba-can*

San. : *Brhamveda Śārngadhara-Caraka*

Auth. : Kun-phan bdud-rtsi byin (Sarvahitāmētadatta)

(14) Tib. : *'Phags-yul dbus-'gyur Ma-thū-ra'i rgyal-rig kyi sman-pa Ra-ghu-nā-tha'i gdams-pa*

San. : *Aryadeśa Māgadha Māthura Kṣatriya bhiṣak Raghunāthanāmāmnāya*

Auth. : Raghunātha.

Medical Works in Noncanonical Literature

In addition to the above mentioned medical works in the Tanjur scriptures, there are several works on medicine prevalent in the non-canonical literature of Tibet. The most popular one amongst them is *Rgyud-bźi* or *Amṛtahṛdaya-aṣṭanga* (*anga-aṣṭa*) *guhyopadeśa-tantra*. Because of its importance, popularity and cryptic nature, several commentaries on the whole or parts of this text were composed and are still available in Tibetan.

Nāgārjuna, the Author

The present work *Vaidya-Jīvasūtra* is placed in second position in the list of medical works included in the Tanjur scriptures. Authorship of this work is attributed to Klu-sgrub (Nāgārjuna) or Klu-sgrub sñiṅ-po (Nāgārjunahṛdaya or Nāgārjunagarbha). Who is this Nāgārjuna, whether he is same as Nāgārjuna-pāda, when did he compose this work and whether he is the same as the propounder of Mādhyamika philosophy of Mahāyāna Buddhism is a subject of hot-debate among the scholars of Indology and Tibetology. In the Tanjur scriptures, the authorship of 122 works is attributed to Nāgārjuna, the authorship of six works is attributed to Nāgārjunahṛdaya (garbha) and that of only one work is attributed to Nāgārjunpāda. The authorship of one such work in the Tanjur is attributed to Kṛṣṇa Nāgārjuna. Use of the terms '*pāda*', '*hṛdaya*' or '*garbha*' as suffix to a name with respect is also common in the tradition. In the ayurvedic tradition of India, authorship of several works on Iatro-chemistry or *Rasaśāstra* and medicine are attributed to Nāgārjuna. Authors entitled to an opinion believe in the existence of four different Nāgārjunas as follows:

(1) Nāgārjuna, the Buddhist philosopher and propounder of Mādhyamika philosophy in Mahāyāna Buddhism. He was born as a brahmin in South India and initially lived a luxurious life with his mystic and magic performances. Later he became a Buddhist. Hiuan-tsang mentions him as a contemporary of the poet Aśvaghoṣa and according to *Rājataranngiṇi* he was a contemporary of Kaniṣka. According to the tradition, he was a friend of the King Śātavāhana who built a monastery for him at Śrīparvata. He probably lived between the 1st and 2nd Century A.D.

(2) Nāgārjuna the Tantric scholar. He belonged to seventh or eighth Cent. A.D.

(3) Nāgārjuna, the author of alchemy and *Rasaśāstra.* He was also known as Siddha Nāgārjuna.

(4) Nāgārjuna, the author of several medical works. He was the redactor of *Suśruta saṃhitā.* According to some scholars, he was the disciple of Bhāskara, and author of works like *Yogaratnamālā.* He flourished before 1240 A.D.

That Nāgārjuna, the author of this and many other works was a Buddhist or at least he was held in high esteem by the Tibetan scholars, is beyond any doubt because of the inclusion of his works in the Tanjur scriptures. Since the original Sanskrit version of this work is no more extant, it is very difficult to get any additional information about this author.

In the Tanjur scriptures, usually the names of the translators or/and revisors are given.But in the case of the present work, such information is not furnished. This need not lead one to believe that the work was originally in Tibetan and not a translated work from original Sanskrit because of the clear statement made in this regard in the beginning of the text.

Positive Health in other Works

Descriptions of positive health and measures for the prevention of diseases are also available in several other religious scriptures and noncanonical literature. In the *Rgyud-bźi*, a mention of which is already made before, such descriptions are available in detail in the following Chapters of *Bśad-pa'i rgyud* or *Ākhyāta tantra* (Explanatory-text) which constitutes its second part.

Chapter-13

Tibetan : Ñin re bźin *rgyun du spyod pa'i le'u*

Sanskrit : *Dinacaryādhyāya*

English : Chapter on regimens for different parts of the day.

Chapter-14

Tib. : Dus su *spyod pa'i le'u*

Sans. : *Ṛtucaryādhyāya*

Eng. : Chapter on regimens for different seasons.

Chapter-15

Tib. : *Gnas skabs kyi spyod lam bstan pa'i le'u*

San. : *Avasthāviśeṣacaryopadeśādhyāya*

Eng. : Chapter on regimens for different situations.

Chapter-16

Tib. : *Zas kyi tshul śes par bya ba'i le'u*

San. : *Āhāravidhivijñānīyādhyāya*

Eng. : Chapter on modes of taking food.

Chapter-17

Tib. : *Kha zas bsdam pa'i le'u*

Sans. : *Āhāraniyamādhyāya.*

Eng. : Chapter on dietatic rules.

Chapter-18

Tib. : *Kha zas bsruṅ ba zas tshod ran par bza' pa'i le'u*

Sans. : *Annarakṣāmātrāśitīyādhyāya*

Eng. : Chapter on protection and quantity of food.

Chapter-19

Tib. : *Ro daṅ źu rjes bstan pa'i le'u*

San. : *Rasavipākopadeśādhyāya*

Eng. : Chapter on the description of tastes and *vipāka* (taste that emerges after digestion)

Chapter-20

Tib. : *Sman gyi nus pa bstan pa'i le'u*

San. : *Auṣadhaviryopadeśādhyāya*

Eng. : Chapter describing the potency of drugs and food-ingredients.

Similar descriptions are available in some of the important Ayurvedic classics as follows:

Caraka-saṃhitā (*Sūtra* 1, 5-7, 25-27)

Suśruta-saṃhitā (*Sūtra* 6, 15, 20, 35, 36, 40, 42)

Aṣṭāṅga-hṛdaya (*Sūtra* 1-13)

Aṣṭāṅga-saṃgraha (*Sūtra* 1, 3-11, 17-20, 23)

Metaphoric Tree

In the *Rgyud-bźi*, all the basic concepts of medicine are metaphorically described in the form of a tree with three roots, nine trunks, 47 branches, 224 leaves, two flowers and three fruits. The basic concepts with regard to the preservation and promotion of positive health and prevention of diseases are includes in the first root (out of the three in total) having two trunks, twelve branches and 88 leaves. The two flowers of this metaphoric tree are:

(1) *Nad med pa* or *vyādhi mukti* (Prevention of diseases, and pres ervation and promotion of positive health)

(2) *Tshe riṅ* or *dīrghāyus* (Promotion of longevity)

The three fruits of this metaphoric tree are:

(1) *Chos* or *dharma* (Endowment of religious virtues)

(2) *Nor* or *artha* (Wealth)

(3) *Bde* or *sukha* or *kama* (Satisfaction of worldly desires).

Lus or Deha-Prakṛti

As has been mentioned before, all the physiological functions of the body are controlled by three factors, viz., *rluṅ* or *vāyu*, *mkhris pa* or *pitta* and *bad kan* or *kapha*. Taken together, these three factors are called *nad* or *ñes pa* (*doṣa* in Ayurveda). When in a state of equilibrium, they help in the maintenance of health and any disturbance in their harmoneous state leads to disease and decay of the body. In practice, it is very difficult to find a person who is possessed with all these three factors in an absolute state of equilibrium. Right at the time of conception when the zygote is formed by the union of the sperm and ovum, there is every possibility of these three elements getting disturbed. Such a disturbance might be in the sperm or ovum or in the womb of the mother. This disturbance is likely to be intensified by the food, drinks and regimens of the mother and by the effects of the environment. If these disturbances cross a limit, then there will be no conception. If however, these disturbances are within limits, then the child born is affected because of the influence of these disturbances, and certain characteristic features are manifested. This is called *lus* or *prakṛti* (physical constitution). On the basis of these characteristic features individuals are divided into seven broad categories - each one of them bearing some specific physical and mental traits. An individual should be examined by the physician to ascertain the type or *deha prakṛti* he possesses and only thereafter, measures in the form of diet, drinks and regimens should be prescribed to keep him healthy. Such persons are prone to certain diseases in their life period. But if they habitually take recourse to these prescriptions and prohibitions, then they remain free from these ailments. Even for the treatment of their diseases, persons having different *lus* or *deha prakṛti* need different types of medicines and therapies even if they are afflicted by the same type of disease.

Yul or Deśa

The second factor which affect the individual is the *yul* or *deśa* (place of habitation). The dry and cold place normally causes aggravation of *rluṅ* or *vāyu*, the hot place normally causes aggravation of *mkhris pa* or *pitta*, and a water-logged wet and cold place causes aggravation of *bad kan* or *kapha.* People inhabiting such places are prone to the attack of certain diseases in the natural course. To keep them healthy, they should resort to certain types of diet, drinks and regimens. Ailments of such persons need some specific types of medicines and therapies.

Dus or Kāla

The third natural factor which afflict a person is the *dus* or *kāla* (temporal factor). This includes the seasonal changes and the various changes, the body and mind of the individual undergo during different parts of the day, night, meal time and span of life. If such changes are within limits then the life-force (*prāṇa*) of an individual is capable of overcoming their adverse effects. If however, this limit is crossed, then the person is afflicted with diseases. The physician should be acquainted with such likely changes in the individual during different seasons, during different parts of the day and night, different phases of food-digestion and during different phases of the life, and prescribe suitable measures both for the prevention and cure of diseases.

The above mentioned three natural factors, viz., lus or d*eha prakṛti* (physical constitution), *yul* or *deśa* (place of habitation) and *dus* or *kāla* (temporal factors) which bring about changes in the equilibrium of *rluṅ* or *vāyu*, *mkris pa* or *pitta* and *bad kan* or *kapha* during the normal course are described in this work, of course in brief. Their adverse effects are to be counteracted with the help of different types of drugs, diet, drinks and regimens. To ascertain which of these ingredients of diet, etc., will be appropriate, it is necessary to know the basic composition of the body and ingredients of food, etc.

Basic Elements in Body

As has been mentioned before, the body of the individual (micro-cosm) is the replica of the universe (macro-cosm). Both the body and the universe are composed of five basic elements called *'byuṅ po chen po* or *mahābhūta.* These are (1) *sa* or *pṛthvī mahābhūta,* (2) *chu* or *jala mahābhūta,* (3) *me* or *agni mahābhūta,* (4) *rluṅ* or *vāyu mahābhūta,* and (5) *nam mkha'* or *ākāśa mahābhūta.* To translate these terms as earth, water, fire, air and ether or sky respectively is likely to lead to misinterpretation of this subtle philosophical concept; hence avoided. In Tibetan medicine, only the first four elements are recognised to take part in the creation of the body and the universe. The variations in *lus* or *deha prakṛti, yul* or *deśa* and *dus* or *kāla* are reflected by the changes of these basic elements in the body and to overcome them it is necessary to supplement the body with appropriate quantity of these elements in the form of food, etc.

In actual practice, determination of these basic elements in the body and ingredients of food, etc., is difficult for a common physician. Therefore, these basic elements of the body are described in the form of *nad* or *ñes pa* (*doṣa*) and from their manifested signs and symptoms, a physician can easily ascertain the status of these basic elements in the body. They represent various basic elements in the body as follows:

	Ñes pa or Doṣa	*'Byuṅ po chen po* or *Mahābhautic* composition
(1)	*Rluṅ* or *Vāyu doṣa*	*Rluṅ* or *Vāyu mahābhūta* (according to Ayurveda, *ākāśa mahābhūta* also takes part, in addition)
(2)	Mkhris pa or *Pitta*	*Me* or *Agni mahābhūta*
(3)	*Bad kan* or *Kapha*	*Sa* or *Pṛthvī mahābhūta* and *Chu* or *Jala Mahābhūta.*

In practice, it is convenient and easy to determine the increase or dicrease of the five basic elements in the body through the manifested signs and symptoms of these three types of *ñes pa* or *doṣa.*

Basic Elements in Food and Drugs

The increased or decreased basic elements in the body are to be corrected by decreasing or increasing them respectively through the administration of various types of food, drinks, regimens and drugs. For convenience and practical utility, the *mahābhautika* composition of these ingredients of food, etc., are described in the form of *ro* or *rasa* (taste), *yon tan* or *guña* (attributes), *nus pa* or *vīrya* (potency), and *zu rjes* or *vipāka* (taste that emerges after digestion). Of these, the first one i.e. taste is of primary importance as all the remaining three are directly or indirectly dependant upon it. These are six in number. The *mahābhautika* composition of a substance which gives rise to these six types of tastes is as follows:

Taste of a Substance	Mahābhautika Composition of the Substance
(1) *Mṅar* or *Madhura* (Sweet)	*Sa* or *Pṛthvī mahābhūta* and *Chu* or *Jala mahābhūta*
(2) *Skyur* or *Amla* (Sour)	*Sa* or *Pṛthvī mahābhūta* and *Me* or *Agni mahābhūta*
(3) *Lan tshwa* or *Lavaṇa* (*Saline taste*)	*Chu* or *Jala mahābhūta* and *Me* or Agni *mahābhūta*
(4) *Tsha ba* or *Kaṭu* (Pungent)	*Me* or *Agni mahābhūta* and *Rluṅ* or *Vāyu mahābhūta*
(5) *Kha ba* or *Tikta* (Bitter)	*Chu* or *Jala mahābhūta* and *Rluṅ* or *Vayu mahābhūta* (*Vāyu* and ākāśa *mahābhūta* according to Ayurveda)
(6) *Bska ba* or *Kaṣāya* (Astringent taste)	*Sa* or *Pṛthvī mahābhūta* and Rluṅ or *Vāyu mahābhūta*

Thus, by examining the condition of *ñes pa* or *doṣa* (through the manifested signs and symptoms), one can easily ascertain the state (increase or decrease) of the basic elements in the body. To correct, this imbalanced state (disturbance in the equilibrium) one can choose the appropriate substance by ascertaining the *Mahābhautika* composition through its taste. Therefore, the nature and effects of these various types of *ro* or *rasa* (taste) are described in this work.

Spyod lam or Regimens

Keeping the above principles in view, regimens for different seasons (*Ṛtu caryā*), different parts of the day (*Dina caryā*) and different parts of the night (*Rātri caryā*) are also described in this text.

Conduct

Since the three types of *ñes pa* or *doṣa* in the body are controlled by three mental factors, viz., *'dod chags* or *kāma* (passion), *źe sdaṅ* or *krodha* (anger or hatred) and *gti mug* or *moha* (illusion), along with physical factors, one should control his mind to be healthy. These mental factors are also described in this text.

Suppression of Natural Urges

Man and other animals share four common traits, viz., (1) *āhāra* or food, (2) *nidrā* or sleep, (3) *bhaya* or fear for external injury and (4) *maithuna* or urge for sex. The only distinctive feature of man (over other animals) is his developed mental faculties or consciousnes (the power to distinguish between right and wrong things). But this distinctive feature has been misused, and the man keeps himself away from the nature. In the pretext of manners and courtesy, he has imposed several restrictions upon himself. One important feature of these inhibitions is the suppression of natural urges (*vega rodha*) which gives rise to several maladies. This has also been explained in this text.

Mutually Contradictory Food

Certain types of food and drinks may be individually useful. But when these are combined together or processed in a particular way, then they produce adverse effects on the body and mind of the individual. Such mutually contradictory food and drinks (*viruddha-annapāna*) are also described in this work.

Duties in Different Stages of Life

Salvation or the absolute freedom from the worldly miseries is the ultimate aim of human beings, and with this aim in view, on should lead a disciplined way of living during different stages of his life. He has to perform certain duties for the welfare of himself, his family, the society and the country during different stages of his life. These duties are also explained in this work.

Brief Nature of Description

What is explained in this text is only an outline of the measures to be adopted by an individual for the preservation and promotion of positive health as well as prevention of diseases. For details, one should collect information scattared in the religious scriptures and noncanonical literature of Tibet and India. If one sincerely desires to provide good health care to the suffering humanity, the commercial aspect of it should be ignored and the measures prescribed in the Traditional medicines of Tibet and India, among others, should be critically studied and adopted. These Traditional systems represent accumulated experience of centuries and a Scientist should not treat them as untouchable. These traditional systems do not represent healthy measures only for the people inhabiting in these specific countries. These are of universal nature and depending upon the social habits and cultural traits of different other countries, necessary modifications can be made in these prescriptions and prohibitions. In this connection, one should keep in view the following statement of Caraka:

"A wise person considers the entire universe as his preceptor. It is only a fool who finds enemies in it. Therefore, a wise person should properly examine and learn even from his so called enemies, such instructions as would endow him with bliss, fame, longevity and nourishment, promote his utility among people, and adopt them in his life."

(*Caraka saṃhitā* : *Vimāna* 8 : 14)

At the end, we share the sentiments of the great saints, philosopher and medical author Klu-sgrub (Nāgārjuna) expressed at the end of his work Sbyor-ba *rgya-pa* (*Yoga-śataka*) as follows:

Yon tan chag can sbyor-ba rgya-pa brjod pa yis /

Bsod nams bla na med pa bdag gis gaṅ thob pa /

De yis rnam pa sna tshogs nad kyi gzir gyur ba /

Mtha' yas 'gro ba rnams kyi nad ni med gyur cig /

गुणाधिकं योगशतं निबध्य

प्राप्तं मया पुण्यमनुत्तमं यत् ।

नानाप्रकारामयनीडभूतं

कृत्स्नं जगत् तेन भवत्वरोगम् ॥

"By the merits par excellence accrued to the author by the composition of *Sbyor-ba rgya pa*, let the universe which is the abode of various types diseases be free from them."

We shall consider our endeavour eminently rewarded even if an iota of this desire is achieved through this work.

Sman 'tsho-ba'i—mdo bźugs //
वैद्य जीव सूत्र विहार (विहरतिस्म).

This work contains Sman 'tsho ba'i mdo (1)
(Vaidya-Jiva-Sūtra)

This is the title of the work. The title in the N & P provides additional information regarding the author of this work, namely Nagarjuna. Whether he is the real author or the work is just attributed to him just to emphasise its authenticity is matter of controversy. Similar is the case of many other works included in the Tanjur and Kanjur scriptures.

Rgya gar skad du Dzī-ba-sū-tra Bod skad du Sman-'tsho-ba'i mdo //
संस्कृत भाषा जीव सूत्र भोट भाषा मन्-छो-वइ-दो (2)
(तिब्बतीय)

In the Sanskrit language this work [was] known as *Jīva-Sūtra*. In the Tibetan language, this [will be] called *Sman 'tsho ba'i mdo*.

Translation of the Tibetan title is *Vaidya-Jīva-Sūtra.* In the original Sanskrit title the term '*Vaidya*' is missing. Works with either of these two titles and with or without the authorship of Nāgārjuna are no more extant in Sanskrit language.

Bam po gcig pa //
भाग प्रथम (3)

This is the first section of the work.

Invocation

Thams cad mkhyen pa la   phyag 'tshal lo //
सर्वज्ञ   नमस्कार   (4)

I bow before the Omniscient One (Lord Buddha).

Sman pa'i mchog   ste   ñon mons   nad   sel   de la   phyag[2] 'tshal   nas //
भिषक्   श्रेष्ठ   क्लेश   रोग   हारी   नमस्   (5)

I bow before the Best among the Physicians (Lord Buddha) who cures mental and physical maladies.

Sarvajña or Omniscient and *Bhiṣak-śreṣṭha* or Best of Physicians are the epithets of Lord Buddha. Often these words and their versions in other languages are used in noun form to mean Lord Buddha himself. Offering prayer or total surrender to him in the beginning of a religious or secular work is a must according to the Buddhist tradition.

This auspicious invocation helps the author or preacher to complete his work without any physical, mental or spiritual inhibition. This invocation also helps the student to successfully complete his study and not to leave the training half the way because of hindrances. In addition, this helps the follower of the tradition to achieve the objective (in the present case to achieve good health).

Traditionally, such auspicious invocations are made in the beginning and at the end, and sometime, at the middle of the text. These are either scribed in the text or just brought to the memory at the time of beginning the writing, preaching or study.

'Phags pa'i   brtul źugs   draṅ sroṅ   ma gtogs   skyes bu   blo ldan pas //
आर्य   मुनि   ऋषि   व्यतिरिक्त   पुरूष   मतिमान्   (6)

Rluṅ   mkhris   bad kan   gsum daṅ   'phrod   spyad   bag bya   spyod lam gyis //
वायु   पित्त   कफ   त्रय   सात्म्य   उपभोग   आहार   विहार   (7)

Mi lus 'di thob don yod 'tsho ba'i don tsam bstan par bya //
मानव शरीर एतत् प्राप्त अर्थ युक्त आयुस् अर्थ किंचित् उपदेश कृत (8)

With the exception of noble saints and sages, for all others, good health is the objective of [holding] the human body and process of living. To maintain this health, and in order to have a purposeful living of this human body which is obtained [by us], the three [basic elements], viz., *rluṅ* (*vāyu*), *mkhris pa* (*pitta*) and *bad kan* (*kapha*), wholesome enjoyments and diet as well as regimens will be described [in this work].

'Dod khro gti mug gsum las rluṅ mkhris bad kan gsum srid de //
काम क्रोध मोह त्रय वायु पित्त कफ त्रय नियमन (9)

Rluṅ (*vāyu*), *mkhris pa* (*pitta*) and *bad kan* (*kapha*), these three are governed by (originate from) three sources, viz., *'dod* (*kāma* or passion), *khro* (*krodha* or anger) and *ti mug* (*moha* or illusion) [respectively].

Lus yul dus la sogs pa kun daṅ bde bcas dbaṅ bskyur źes //
देह देश काल इत्यादि सर्व सुख सह नियमन इति (10)

Draṅ sroṅ chen pos gsuṅs phyir de yi khyad par mdor bstun[3] nas //
महर्षि कथन हेतु तत् विशेषतः समासतः (11)

Tshul rtags[4] zas daṅ gnas dpyad[5] dgoṅs pa ñi tshe 'dir brjod pa //
चर्या लक्षण अन्न स्थान परीक्षा अभिप्राय प्रदेश एतत् कथन (12)

Happiness is subjected to different changes in the body, place of habitation and seasons, for which, on the lines of the instructions of great sages, topics relating to conduct, constitution, food and place of habitation are specially described here for the purpose of examination (investigation).

LUS (DEHA PRAKṚTI OR PHYSICAL CONSTITUTION)

Characteristic features of the body including mind vary from individual to individual. In ayurveda, this is called *deha prakṛti* or just *prakṛti*. These variations are caused because of the condition of *ñes pas* (*doṣas*) in the womb of the mother at the time of conception (union of the sperm and ovum). Broadly, these variations are grouped into seven categories, viz., (1) rluṅ predominant (*vāta prakṛti*), (2) *mkhris pa predominant* (*pitta prakṛti*), (3) *bad kan* predominant (*kapha prakṛti*), (4) - (6) predominance of two of the above mentioned elements and (7) equilibrium of all the three elements. If *rluṅ*, *mkhris pa* and *bad kan* are all in an aggravated state, then there will be no conception.

Predominance of these elements produces a characteristic physical and mental trait in the individual which persists for the entire life period and any change in these traits or characteristic features are indicative of bad prognosis or are signs of imminent death.

These characteristic features help the physician both in the prevention and cure of diseases. Each group has a tendency to be affected by certain selected diseases and if proper precaution is taken in the form of diet and regimens, then such diseases could be easily prevented. Appearance of certain diseases in these groups result in serious repercussions. Therefore, the physician should be extra cautious to treat such ailments.

Lus rtsub skems sems rgod tshig maṅ graṅ rluṅ gi mi //
देह रुक्ष कृश मनस् विचलित वाक् अधिक शीत वायु मानव (13)

Ununctuousness and thinness of the body, agitated mind, garrulousness and cold-feeling—these are the characteristic features of the person having predominance of *rluṅ* (*vāta prakṛti*).

Dmar ser blo rno khro la drod che dri can mkhris pa'i mi //
रक्त पीत बुद्धि तीक्ष्ण क्रोध उष्ण अधिक गन्ध युक्त पित्त मनुष्य (14)

Red and yellow colour [of the body], sharp intelligence, excessive anger and heat in the body and excessively bad smell coming out of the body - these are the characteristic features of the person having predominance of *mkhris pa* (*pitta prakṛti*).

Dkar snum tshig G'yuṅ lci la drod chuṅ gñid chuṅ bad kan mi //
श्वेत स्निग्ध वाक् मंगल गुरु उष्ण अल्प निद्रा अल्प कफ मानव (15)

Whiteness, ununctuousness, less of (auspicious) talk, heaviness (deep voice), less of heat and less of sleep—these are the characteristic features of the person having predominance of *bad kan* (*kapha prakṛti*).

The person of *kapha prakṛti* normally sleeps more. Therefore, the more appropriate reading of *gñid chuṅ* should have been *gñid maṅ*.

Gñis daṅ gsum du 'dres pa yaṅ ni de las śes par bya //
द्वि त्रय मिलित यदि तथा ज्ञान करण (16)

If two or three of these elements, viz., *rluṅ* (*vāyu*), *mkhris pa* (*pitta*) and *bad kan* (*kapha*) jointly become predominant, then their respective characteristic features (described above) will be together manifested.

The above description pertains to the remaining four of the seven groups in total of physical constitution. These are the characteristic features (*prakṛtis*) caused by the predominance of (1) *rluṅ* and *mkhris pa*, (2) *mkhris pa* and *bad kan*, (3) *rluṅ* and *bad kan* and (4) *rluṅ*, *mkhris pa* and *bad kan*.

In the last group, all the three elements remain in a state of equilibrium because their aggravated state in the uterus at the time of conception and therefore in the zygote (embryo) is not possible. In such a state when all these three elements are in an aggravated stage, there is no possibility of conception.

6

Rgan daṅ dar daṅ byis pa rim gyis lta źiṅ śes par bya //
वृद्ध युवा बाल यथाक्रम दर्शन ज्ञान करण (17)

[Like that, predominance of *rluṅ* (*vāyu*), *mkhris pa* (*pitta*) and *bad kan* (*kapha*) takes place] in the old age, in youth and in children respectively. This should be seen and ascertained.

Along with the knowledge of physical constitution (*lus* or *deha prakṛti*) it is necessary to know the predominance of *rlu◊* etc., in different stages of life. In old age, *rlu◊* (*vāyu*) is generally predominant, in the youth *mkhris pa* (*pitta*) is predominant and in infancy, *bad kan* (*kapha*) is predominant. Therefore, proper examination of the age of the patient is essential for the maintenance and promotion of positive health and prevention as well as cure of diseases.

YUL (DEŚA OR PLACE OF HABITATION)

In addition to body, the place of habitation is also dominated by *rluṅ* (*vāyu*), etc. Determination of these characteristic features is also useful for the maintenance and promotion of positive health and prevention as well as cure of diseases.

Ṅad can graṅ ba rluṅ gi yul te tsha gduṅ mkhris pa'i sa //
वातल शीतल वायु देश उष्ण तप्त पित्त भूमि (18)

Rlan can snum bag bad kan yul te 'dres pa de las brtag //
आर्द्र स्निग्ध कफ देश मिश्र परीक्षा (19)

The airy (windy) and cold region is the land of *rluṅ (vāyu)*; the hot region is the land of *mkhris pa* (*pitta*); and the region with humidity as well as unctuousness is the land of *bad kan* (*kapha*). The mixed regions will have mixed characteristic features. Thus, the nature of the land should be examined.

In the land of *rluṅ*, generally the inhabitants are more afflicted with diseases caused by *rluṅ* (*vāyu*). For the prevention of these diseases, the inhabitants should habitually use food and adopt regimens which are alleviators of *rluṅ* (*vāyu*). Hot and unctuous food and regimens are useful for such inhabitants. Similarly, the inhabitants of *mkhris pa* (*paittika*) type of land should use cooling food and regimens, and those of *bad kan* (*kaphaja*) land should use dry and ununctuous food and regimens.

DUS (RLUṄ, etc, IN DIFFERENT PARTS OF DAY & NIGHT AND IN DIFFERENT SEASONS)

The very process of living makes the tissue elements in the body to grow, to get stabilised and to undergo the process of decay in different phases of the life. Similarly, as a natural manifestation of this biological phenomenon, *rluṅ* (*vāyu*), *mkhris pa* (*pitta*) and *bad kan* (*kapha*) get aggravated during different parts of the day and night. This phenomena become explicit in the form of accumulation, aggravation and alleviation during different seasons. This disturbance in the harmony of elements generally takes place within certain limits and the healthy body adjusts itself to these variations without any difficulty. But, if the body is not in good shape then a person is likely to fall victim to diseases because of these fluctuations. For the maintenance and promotion of positive health, and for the prevention and cure of diseases adequate care should be taken in the form of appropriate food, drinks, regimens and even medicines during these periods of natural disturbance of harmony among elements.

Naṅ par srod ni bad kan tho raṅs phyi dro rluṅ gi dus //
प्रातः सायं कफ प्रत्युष अपराह्ण वायु काल (20)

Ñi ma phyed daṅ nam phyed mkhris pa'i dus yin śes par bya //
मध्याह्न मध्यरात्रि पित्त काल ज्ञान करण (21)

Morning and evening (early part of the night) are the times for [the aggravation of] *bad kan* (*kapha*). Dawn (last part of the night) and the after-noon are the times for [the aggravation of] *rluṅ* (*vāyu*). Mid-day and the mid-night are the times for [the aggravation of] *mkhris pa* (*pitta*). This, one should know.

7

Dpyid na bad kan ldaṅ ste dbyar stod rluṅ gsog ston mkhris ldaṅ //
वसन्त कफ प्रकोप ग्रीष्म वायु संचय शरत् पित्त प्रकोप (22)

8 9

Dbyar smad rluṅ ldaṅ mkhris gsog dgun stod dgun smad bad kan gsog //
प्रावृट् वायु प्रकोप पित्त संचय हेमन्त शिशिर कफ संचय (23)

Ston ni rluṅ źi dgun stod mkhris źi dbyar smad bad kan źi //
शरत् वायु प्रशम हेमन्त पित्त प्रशम प्रावृट् कफ प्रशम (24)

Bad kan (*kapha*) gets aggravated during the spring season. *Rluṅ* (*vāyu*) gets accumulated in the first part of summer. *Mkhris pa* (*pitta*) gets aggravated in the autumn.

Rluṅ (*vāyu*) gets aggravated in the late summer. *Mkhris pa* (*pitta*) gets accumulated in the late summer. In the early winter and late winter *bad kan* (*kapha*) gets accumulated.

In the autumn *rluṅ* (*vāyu*) gets alleviated. In the early winter *mkhris pa* (*pitta*) gets alleviated. In the late summer *bad kan* (*kapha*) gets alleviated.

Depending upon the position of the sun, different parts of the globe experience different seasons during different periods of the year. Ayurvedic classics of ancient India describe these seasonal variations in two different ways—one for the manifestation of *rasas* (tastes) in ingredients of food, drinks, and medicines and the other for the description of variations or changes in the states of *doṣas*, viz., *vāyu* (*rluṅ*), *pitta* (*mkhris pa*) and *kapha* (*bad kan*). This latter type of classification is relevant in the present context.

In view of the difference in the geographical position, Tibet has different types of seasons each experienced in different calender months. To explain the condition (accumulation, aggravation and alleviation) of *rluṅ*, *mkhris pa* and *bad kan* in different periods of the year, it has been divided into six seasons in a slightly different manner. The accumulation, etc., of *rluṅ* (*vāyu*), *mkhris pa* (*pitta*) and *bad kan* (*kapha*) are given in the following table:

Table Showing the Condition of *Rluṅ*, etc., in Different Seasons

Name of the Season				*Condition of Ñes pa*		
	Tibetan	*English*	*Sanskrit*	*Rluṅ*	*Mkhris pa*	*Bad kan*
(1)	*Dbyar stod*	Summer (early)	griṣma	accumu-lation		alleviation according to ayurvedic texts
(2)	*Dbyar smad*	Summer (later part)	*prāvṛt*	aggrava-tion	accumu-lation	alleviation according to Tibetan medicine
(3)	*Ston*	Autumn	*śarat*	alleviation	aggravation	accumulation
(4)	*Dgun stod*	Winter (early)	*hemanta*			accumulation
(5)	*Dgun smad*	Winter (later part)	*śiśira*			accumulation
(6)	*Dpyid*	spring	*vasanta*			aggravation

The description, in this connection, in the Tibetan text is almost similar to that available in ayurvedic texts except the portion describing the alleviation of *bad kan* (*kapha*). There appears to be an error in the 24th line in as much as instead of *dbyar smad* meaning "late summer" it should read *dbyar stod*".

RO (RASAS OR TASTES) AND RLUN, ETC.

The effects of the ingredients of drug, diet and drinks are primarily determined on the basis of their tastes which are six in number. These are sweet, sour, saline, pungent, bitter and astringent. Modern science does not accept pungent and astringent as real tastes because of the absence of specific taste-buds in the tongue for their perception. None the less, Ayurveda and Tibetan medicine have categorically recognised all these six tastes and described the properties of various ingredients accordingly.

10

Lus yul dus dag brjod nas ro drug khad par mdor bstan pa //

देह देश काल कथन अनन्तर रस षट् विशेषतः संक्षेपतः उपदिष्ट (25)

Having completed the description of *lus* (*deha* or body), *yul* (*deśa* or place of habitation) and *dus* (*kāla* or time incuding day, night & seasons) [with reference to their relationship with *rlun*, *mkhris pa* and *bad kan*], now the effects of six tastes will be specially described in brief.

Sweet Taste

11

Mnar kun bsil te bad kan skyed de rlun mkhris sel byed na //

मधुर सर्व शीतल कफ जनक वायु पित्त शमन कारक (26)

All the ingredients having sweet taste are cooling and they aggravate *bad kan* (*kapha*). In addition, they alleviate *rlun* (*vāyu*) and *mkhris pa* (*pitta*).

Exceptions (Sweet Ingredients having Heating Effect)

Źun mar bu ram sñin gzer gze ma gro dan star ka dro //

घृत गुड ? गोक्षुर गोधुम अक्षोट उष्ण (27)

Some sweet ingredients like ghee, jaggery, *sñin gzer* (?), *gze ma* (*gokṣura* = *Tribulus terrestris*), wheat and *sta rka* (*akṣota* = walnut) are exceptions (to the rule stipulated in the line 26) inasmuch as these are of heating effect.

Exception (Sweet Ingredients having *Bad Kan* Alleviating Property)

Mu ka[12] sbraṅ rtsi[13] skam sa'i śa daṅ nas daṅ bu ram rñiṅ[14] //
मुद्‌ग मधु जांगल मांस यव गुड पुराण (28)

Bad kan sel te ñe śiṅ ram ñe bad kan mi skyed sñoms //
कफ शामक ? नीली कफ न उत्पादक साम्योत्पादक (29)

Some sweet ingredients like *mudga* (*Phaseolus mungo*), honey, meat of animals living in arid zone, barley and old jaggery are also exceptions (to the rule stipulated in the line 26) inasmuch as they alleviate *bad kan* (*kapha*). Similarly, some sweet ingredients like *ñe śiṅ* (?) and *ram ñe (nīlī = Indigofera tinctoria)* do not aggravate *bad kan* but help maintaining its equilibrium.

Pungent Test

Tsha ba dro ste mkhris skye[15] rluṅ daṅ bad kan sel byed na //
कटु उष्ण पित्त कारक वायु कफ शमन कारक (30)

Pungent taste is hot. It aggravates *mkhris pa* (*pitta*) and alleviates *rluṅ* (*vāyu*) and *bad kan* (*kapha*).

Exceptions

Srog chags mkhris pa mkhris sel na le śam ni rluṅ yaṅ skyed[16] //
प्राणि पित्त पित्त शामक मरिच वायु जनक (31)

[Some pungent ingredients are exceptions to the above rule inasmuch as] animal bile alleviates *mkhris pa* (*pitta*) and *na le śam* (*marica* = *Piper nigrum*) aggravate *rluṅ* (*vāyu*).

Sour taste

Skyur kun dro ste mkhris pa skyed[17] ciṅ bad kan rluṅ sel na //
अम्ल सर्व उष्ण पित्त कारक कफ वायु शामक (32)

All sour ingredients are hot, aggravator of *mkhris pa* and alleviator of *bad kan* (*kapha*) and *rluṅ* (*vāyu*).

Exceptions

Skyu ru ra dan bal po se'u ni mkhris pa sel bar byed //
आमलकी दाडिम पित्त शमन कारक (33)

Ku śu mnar ni bsil la dar ba chus bslad mkhris mi skyed //
सेव मधुर शीतल तक्र जल मिश्रित पित्त न कारक (34)

[Some sour ingredients are exceptions to this rule inasmuch as] *skyu ru ra* (*āmalakī=Emblica officinalis*) and pomegranate alleviate *mkhris pa* (*pitta*). Similarly, apple, though sweet [should have been sour] is cooling and buttermilk [though sour] does not aggravase *mkhris pa* (*pitta*).

The term '*ku śu*' is generally used for apple, but it is also used for *nimbu* (lemon). Contextually the term '*skyur*' meaning sour should have appeared in the place of *mnar* meaning sweet in the line 34.

Bitter taste

18

Kha ba bsil te rlun skyed bad kan mkhris pa sel byed na //
तिक्त शीतल वायु वर्धक कफ पित्त शमन कारक (35)

Ingredients having bitter taste are cooling, aggravator of *rlun* (*vāyu*) and alleviator of *bad kan* (*kapha*) and *mkhris pa* (*pitta*).

Exceptions

Śu dag sle tres dro ste 'phrod dan sbyar na rlun yan sel //
वचा गुडूची उष्ण सात्म्य मिश्रित वायु शामक (36)

[Some bitter ingredients are exceptions to this rule inasmuch as] *śu dag* (*vacā = Acorus calamus*) and *sle tres* (*guḍūcī = Tinospora cordifolia*) are hot and wholesome. Added [with other drugs], these drugs alleviate *rlun* (*vāyu*).

Astringent taste

Bska ba kun ni bsil te rluṅ skyed bad kan mkhris sel na //
कषाय सर्व शीतल वायु वर्धक कफ पित्त शामक (37)

All ingredients having astringent taste are cooling. They aggravate *rluṅ* (*vāyu*) and alleviate *mkhris pa* (*pitta*).

Exceptions

19
A ru ra ni ñes pa gsum la gnod mi byed de sñoms //
हरीतकी दोष त्रय दूषण न कारक साम्योत्पादक (38)

20
Chaṅ ran bad kan rluṅ sel maṅ na mkhris pa skyed par byed
मद्य सम्यक् कफ वायु शामक अधिक पित्त। जनन कारक (39)

[Some astringent ingredients are exceptions to this rule inasmuch as] *a ru ra* (*harītakī* = *Terminalia chebula*) does not vitiate the three *ñes* (*doṣas*), [viz., *rluṅ* or *vāyu*, *mkhris pa* or *pitta and bad kan* or *kapha*]. [On the other hand *a ru ra*] promotes their harmony. Similarly, alcohol taken in appropriate quantity alleviates *bad kan* (*kapha*) and *rluṅ* (*vāyu*), and when taken in excess quantity it aggravates *mkhris pa* (*pitta*).

Saline Taste

21
Lan tshwa dro ste rluṅ sel bad kan mkhris pa skyed byed na //
लवण उष्ण वायु शामक कफ पित्त। जनन कारक (40)

Ingredients having saline taste are hot, alleviator of *rluṅ* (*vāyu*) and aggravator of *bad kan* (*kapha*) as well as *mkhris pa* (*pitta*).

Exceptions

22 23
Rgyam tsha lce myaṅ tsha ni mkhris pa la yaṅ gnod mi byed //
सैन्धव स्फुटिका पित्त दुष्टि न कारक (41)

[Some saline ingredients are exceptions to this rule inasmuch as] *rgyam tsha* (*saindhava* = rock-salt) and *lce myaṅ tsha* (*sphuṭikā* = alum) do not vitiate (aggravate) *mkhris pa* (*pitta*).

The following table shows the effects of different *ro* (*rasa* = taste) on *ñes* (*doṣa*), as described in Ayurveda.

RO		*Ñes (doṣa)*	
(rasa or taste)	*rluṅ (vāyu)*	*mkhris pa (pitta)*	*baḋ kan (kapha)*
(1) *Mṅar* (*madhura* or sweet)	*alleviation*	*alleviation*	*aggravation*
(2) *Skyur* (*amla* or sour)	alleviation	aggravation	aggravation
(3) *Lan tshwa* (*lavaṇa* or saline)	alleviation	aggravation	aggravation
(4) *Tsha ba* (*Kaṭu or pungent*)	aggravation	aggravation	alleviation
(5) *Kha ba* (*tikta* or bitter)	*aggravation*	*alleviation*	*alleviation*
(6) *Bska ba* (*kaṣāya* or astringent)	*aggravation*	*alleviation*	*alleviation*

RO (*RASA* OR TASTE) AND *YON TAN* (GUṆA OR ATTRIBUTE)

Ro or tastes are six in number as described before, viz., sweet, sour, saline, pungent, bitter and astringent. (In the text above, these are described in a slightly different order). Philosophically, these are the attributes of substance (*dravya*). But in the context of therapeutics or medical science these are stated to have attributes which are broadly twenty in number, and called *yon tan* (*guṇa*). Eight of these attributes are more potent for which these are called *nus pa* (*vīrya* or potency). Some of these potent attributes are present in *ro* (*rasa* or taste) in different states, viz., more (*uttama*), moderate (*madhyama*) and less (*avara*). This relative preponderance of various attributes in tastes is described here.

Mṅar daṅ bska daṅ lan tshwa gsum yaṅ rim bźin[24] mas lci[25] ste //
मधुर कषाय लवण त्रय क्रमशः अनुलोमन गुरू (42)

Among sweet, astringent and saline tastes the earlier ones are more *mas* (*anulomana* = which causes downward movement of *rluṅ or vāyu*) than the latter ones. Similarly the earlier ones are heavier than the latter ones.

By implication, sweet, astrinent and sour tastes, all these three are *mas* (*anulomana*) and lci (*guru*). But sweet taste is more *mas* and *lci*, astringent taste is moderately *mas* and *lci* and saline taste is less *mas* and *lci*.

Skyur daṅ tsha[26] daṅ kha ba gsum ni de bźin rim[27] źiṅ[28] yaṅ //
अम्ल कटु तिक्त त्रय तथा क्रमशः लघु (43)

Among sour, pungent and bitter tastes, the latter ones are lighter than the former ones.

By implication, sour, pungent and bitter tastes are light in attribute. But bitter is more light, pungent is moderately light and sour is less light.

29

Kha ba bska daṅ lan tshwa gsum yaṅ rim bzin mas rtshub ste //
तिक्त कषाय लवण त्रय क्रमशः अनुलोमन रुक्ष (44)

Among the three tastes, viz., bitter, astringent and saline, the earlier ones are more *mas* (*anulomana* = which cause downward movement of *rluṅ* or *vāyu*) and more ununctuous than the latter ones.

By implication, bitter, astringent and saline tastes are *mas* (*anulomana*) and *rtsu ba* (*rukṣa* or ununctuous). But bitter is more *mas* and *rtsu ba*, astringent is moderately *mas* and *rtsu ba*, and saline is less *mas* and *rtsu ba*.

30 31

Mnar daṅ skyur daṅ tsha ba gsum yaṅ de bzin mar ziṅ 'jam //
मधुर अम्ल कटु त्रय क्रमशः स्निग्ध मृदु (45)

Among the three tastes, viz., sweet, sour and pungent, the earlier ones are more soft and unctuous than the latter ones.

By implication, sweet, sour and pungent tasks are unctuous and soft (*mṛdu*). But sweet is more unctuous and soft, sour is moderately unctuous and soft and pungent is less unctuous and soft.

There appears to be several calligraphic errors in the texts from 42 to 45. Fully aware of these errors we have tried to be faithful to the texts which can be revised after further research work.

The table below gives the relative preponderance of various attributes in different tastes as described in Ayurveda. (*Caraka Saṁhitā* and Vāgbhaṭa's *Aṣṭāṅgahṛdaya*)

Yon tan or *nus pa* (*guṅa or vīrya or attributes*)	more (*uttama*)	moderate (*madhyama*)	less (*avara)*
(1) *Rukṣa* (*rtsu ba* or ununctuousness)	*kaṣāya* or astringent (bska ba)	*kaṭu* or pungent (*tsha ba*)	or *tikta* or bitter (*kha ba*)
(2) *Snigdha* (*mas* or unctuousness)	*madhura* or *sweet* (*mṅar ba*)	*amla or sour* (*skyur ba*)	*lavaṇa or* (*lan tshwa*)
(3) *Uṇa* (*dro* or hot)	*lavaṅa* or sline (*lan tshwa*)	*amla or sour* (*skyur ba*)	*kaṭu* or pungent (*tsha ba*)
(4) *Śīta* (*bśil ba or* cold)	*kaṣāya* or astringent (*bska ba)*[1]	*madhura* or sweet (*mṅar ba)*[2]	*tikta* or bitter (*kha ba*)
(5) *Guru* (lci or heavy)	*madhura* or sweet (*mṅar ba)*	*kaṣāya* or astringent (*bska ba)*	*lavaṇa* or saline (*lan tshwa*)
(6) *Laghu* (*yaṅ* or light)	*tikta* or bitter (*kha ba)*	*kaṭu* or pungent (tsha ba)	*amla* or sour (*skyur ba)*

(1) *Madhura* or sweet (*mṅar ba*) according to *Aṣṭāṅga hṛdaya.*
(2) *Kaṣāya or astringent (bska ba*) according to *Aṣṭāṅga hṛdaya.*

Rluṅ mkhris bad kan gsum ka[32] 'dra ste ñid kyis ñid skyes[33] pas //
वायु पित्त कफ त्रय स्वंय आत्म आत्म जनन (46)

Lus daṅ yul dus zas spyod tshul gcig 'dom na nad ldaṅ ste //
देह देश काल अन्न विहार एक वर्णन रोग कारक (47)

The three [*ñes pa*], viz., *rluṅ* (*vāyu*), *mkhris pa* (*pitta*) and *bad kan* (*kapha*) being themselves aggravated because of physical constitution (*lus*), country of habitation (*yul*), time or seasonal variations (*dus*) and conduct (*spyod tshul*) produce diseases.

Ji ltar mthun par 'phrod sbyar luṅ mkhris bad kan mi ldaṅ phan //
यथा अनुकूल सात्म्य मिश्रित वायु पित्त कफ न कारक हित (48)

De phyir 'phrod daṅ mi 'phrod la sogs tshul bźin 'dir bstan pa //
तदर्थ सात्म्य असात्म्य इत्यादि आचार यथा अत्र उपदिष्ट (49)

Rluṅ (*vāyu*), *mkhris pa* (*pitta*) and *bad kan* (*kapha*) do not get aggravated by the wholesome adoption of the above mentioned factors which is beneficial for good health. Therefore, conducts which are wholesome and unwholesome, etc., [for health] are being explained here accordingly.

Useful and harmful factors for *rluṅ* (*vāyu*)

34

Rluṅ ni mṅar snum lci dro 'phrod de rtsub yaṅ bsil mi ' phrod //
वायु मधुर स्निग्ध गुरू उष्ण सात्म्य रुक्ष लघु शीतल न सात्म्य (50)

For *rluṅ* (*vāyu*) sweet, unctuous, heavy and hot ingredients are useful. [On the other hand], things which are ununctuous, light and cooling are harmful for *rluṅ* (*vāyu*).

Useful and harmful factors for *mkhris pa (pitta)*

35

Mkhris pa kha mṅar bsil daṅ 'phrod de tsha skyur dro mi 'phrod //
पित्त तिक्त मधुर शीतल हितकर कटु अम्ल उष्ण न सात्म्य (51)

For *mkhris pa* (*pitta*), bitter, sweet and cooling things are useful. [On the other hand] things which are pungent, sour and heat producing are harmful for *mkhris pa* (*pitta*).

Useful and harmful factors for *bad kan (kapha)*

36

Bad kan snum lci bsil daṅ mi 'phrod rtsub tsha sphyod daṅ 'phrod //
कफ स्निग्ध गुरू शीतल न हितकर रुक्ष उष्ण चर्या हितकर (52)

For *bad kan* (*kapha*), unctuous, heavy and cooling things are harmful. [On the other hand], ununctuous and hot things (regimens) are useful for *bad kan* (*kapha*).

De bas raṅ gi lus daṅ dus gnas za daṅ 'phrod spyaṅ phyir //
आत्मन् देह काल स्थान अन्न हितकर आचरण हेतु (53)

In order to adopting agreeable time, place and food according to one's own body, [a person] should adopt [the following seasonal regimens.]

REGIMENS FOR DIFFERENT SEASONS
(ṚTU CARYĀ)

Food, drinks and other regimens which are suitable and which are unsuitable for different seasons will now be described. In Ayurveda seasonal classification of the year is attempted in two different ways as given in the table below:

Season according to Caraka 1	*Month according to Hindu Calender*	*Month according to Gregarian Calender*	*Season according to Vāgbhaṭa* [2]
(1) *Grīṣma*	*Vaiśākha*	April-May	
			Grīṣma
(Summer)	*Jyeṣṭha*	May-June	(Summer)
(2) *Prāvṛt*	*Āṣāḍha*	June-July	(Tib. *Dbyar stod)*
(Early rain)	*Śrāvaṇa*	July-August	*Varśa*
			(Rainy season)
(3) *Varṣā*	*Bhādrapada*	August-Sept.	(Tib.Dbyar smad)
(Rainy season)	*Āśvina*	Sept.-Oct.	*Śarat*
			(Autumn)
			(Tib. *Ston)*
(4) *Śarat*	*Kārtika*	Oct.-Nov.	
(Autumn)	*Margaśīrṣa*	Nov.-Dec.	*Hemanta*
			(Early winter)
(5) *Hemanta*	*Pauṣa*	Dec.-Jan.	(Tib. *Dgun stod)*
(Winter)	*Māgha*	Jan.-Feb.	*Siśira*
			(Late winter)
(6) *Vasanta*	*Phālguna*	Feb.-March	(Tib. *Dgun smad)*
(Spring)	*Caitra*	March-April	*Vasanta*
			(Spring)
	[*Vaiśākha*]	April-May	(Tib. *Dpyid)*

(1) *Caraka: Vimāna 8:125 to determine the aggravation, etc., of doṣas.*

(2) *Aṣṭāṅga hṛdaya: Sūtra* 3:1 to explain the manifestation of tastes.

In Tibet, because of typical geogaphical situation, seasons are described differently. The commonly used seasonal classification is given below:

(1) Dpyid (Spring)	zla ra pa	*Phñāguna*	Feb.-March
"	zla 'briṅ po	*Caitra*	March-April
"	zla chuṅ	*Vaiśākha*	April-May
(2) Dbyar (Summer)	zla ra pa	*Jyeṣṭha*	May-June
"	zla 'briṅ po	Āṣāḍha	June-July
"	zla chuṅ	*Śrāvaṇa*	July-August
(3) Ston (Autumn)	zla ra pa	*Bhādrapada*	August-September
"	zla 'briṅ po	*Āśvina*	September-October
"	zla chuṅ	*Kārtika*	October-November
(4) Dgun (Winter)	zla ra pa	Mārgaśira	November-December
"	zla 'briṅ po	*Pauṣa*	December-January
"	zla chuṅ	*Māgha*	January-February

In the present work, seasonal classification as given in Vāgbhaṭa's *Aṣṭāṅga hṛdaya* is followed.

REGIMENS FOR *DPYID* (*SPRING*)

Dpyid zla gñis ni bad kan bskyed dus yin te nad ldaṅ bas //
वसन्त मास द्वय कफ कारक काल रोग उत्पन्न (54)

During the two months of spring, *bad kan* (*kapha*) gets aggravated causing there by diseases.

Therapies

Bad kan draṅ źiṅ bkru sman skyug sman btaṅ źiṅ chu tshan btuṅ //
कफ आकर्षण विरेचन वमन प्रयोग उष्णजल पान (55)

[During spring], for taking out *bad kan* (*kapha*), purgation and emetic therapies should be administered and [the patient should be given hot water to drink.

Food

Gro nas bsreg śa sbraṅ rtsi la sogs rtsub bska yaṅ ba bza' //
गोधुम यव भर्जित मांस मधु इत्यादि रूक्ष कषाय लघु भोजन (56)

[During spring] one should take (eat) wheat, barley, roasted meat, honey, etc., which are ununctuous, astringent and light.

Drinks

Sbraṅ chaṅ rguṅ chaṅ sga[37] chu sbraṅ chu bu ram[38] chaṅ rñiṅ[39] btuṅ //
मध्वासव द्राक्षासव शुण्ठी उदक मधु उदक गुड पुराणमद्य पान (57)

[During spring] one should drink *spraṅ chaṅ (madhvāsava* = alcoholic drink prepared of honey), *rgun chaṅ* (*drākṣāsava* = alcoholic drink prepared of grape), water boiled with ginger, water mixed with honey, jaggery and old wine.

Prohibitions

Mar tshil la sogs snum lci kha ra skyur po tsha phrom dag //
नवनीत वसा इत्यादि स्निग्ध गुरू शर्करा अम्ल लवण ? (58)

Mṅar 'jam skyur na bsil bag yaṅ źiṅ ñin par log mi bya //
मधुर मृदु अल शीतल अन्न दिवानिद्रा न कर्तव्य (59)

[During spring] one should not take butter, fat, etc., which are unctuous and heavy, sugar, sour and salty things, *phrom* (?), and one should avoid sweet, soft, sour, cooling things, and sleep during the day time.

The meaning the terms *skyur po* and *tsha phrom* is not clear. The term *log* means opposite. During the day time one should remain awake. Thus, by implication *ñin par log* means "sleep during day time".

Other Regimens

Chu[40] tshas lus bkru mñe ziṅ[41] lus[42] bskyod bcag bya ci ran bya //
उष्णोदक स्नान अभ्यंग व्यायाम चंक्रमण यथायोग्य कर्तव्य (60)

[During spring] one should take bath in hot water and resort to massage, exercise and walk appropriately.

Habitation

Gnas kyaṅ ha caṅ mi tsha mi graṅ ran dro grib mar 'dug[43] //
स्थान अधिक न उष्ण न शीतल सुखोष्ण छाया विश्राम (61)

[During spring] one should take rest in a place which is neither very hot nor very cold but comfortably warm and in a shady place.

REGIMENS FOR *DBYAR STOD* (EARLY SUMMER)

44

Dbyar stod zla gñis mar 'bri dus yin ñal po drag śul spaṅ //
ग्रीष्म मास द्वय आदान काल व्यवाय व्यायाम त्याग (62)

The two months of the summer season constitute *mar 'bri dus* (*ādāna kāla* or the time of absorption when the vitality of the body is reduced because of excessive heat of the sun). During this season sexual intercourse and vigorous exercise should be avoided.

Ṅal dub mi bya bag 'bras o'ma mar sar śa dag bza' //
श्रम न कर्तव्य शाल्यन्न दुग्ध नवनीत मांस भोजन (63)

[During summer], one should not get fatigued and he should eat boiled rice milk, butter and meat.

Bu ram tshil ni cuṅ zad bza' ste chaṅ ñuṅ yaṅ ba btuṅ //
गुड वसा अल्प अन्न भोजन मद्य अल्प लघु पान (64)

[During summer], one should eat less of molasses and animal fat and he should drink light type of alcohol in small quantity.

45

O' ma bskol graṅ kha ras btab daṅ dar ba 'thuṅs na phan //
दुग्ध शृत शीत शर्करा युक्त तक्र पान हित (65)

[During summer], one should drink boiled and cooled milk added with sugar and should also drink butter-milk.

46 47

Lan tshwa skyur źiṅ na le śam la sogs pa tsha skyur spaṅ //
लवण अम्ल मरिच इयादि उष्ण (कटु) अम्ल त्याग (66)

[During summer], one should avoid saline and sour thing and such other hot and sour things like *na le śam* (*marica = Piper nigrum*), etc.

48

Chu 'jam tsam gyis lus bkru sgra sñan mñan źiṅ gdags //
जल सुखोष्ण शरीर स्नान संगीत सभक्ति श्रवण परिधान (67)

[During summer] one should take bath in luke-warm water and hear sweet songs.

This text has only 11 words where as previous and latter texts have 13 words each. Perhaps two words are missing from this text for which the implication of the last word *'gdags'* is not clear.

49

Char par reg bya ñin par tsog bur gñid kyis log na phan //
वर्षा स्पर्शकरण दिवा आसन शयन हितकर (68)

[During summer], if it rains, then one should expose himself to rain, and during day time sitting (resting) and sleeping are useful.

50

Gnas kyaṅ ser bu drag po'i ṅad med dro min bsil bar 'dug //
आवास करका वात्या रहित अनुष्ण शीतल निवास (69)

[During summer], one should reside in a house which is protected from hail-stone and tornado, and which is not hot but cool.

REGIMENS FOR DBYAR SMAD (LATE SUMMER)

Dbyar smad zla ba gñis na mkhris pa gsog[51] śiṅ[52] rluṅ ldaṅ ste //
प्रावृट्‌ मास द्वय पित्त संचय वायु प्रकोप (70)

During the two months of late-summer, *mkhris pa* (*pitta*) gets accumulated and *rluṅ* (*vāyu*) gets aggravated in the body.

Phyi rol tsha la lus kyi naṅ graṅ[53] nad gsum g'yos[54] pas na //
वाह्य उष्ण देह आभ्यन्तर शीत रोग त्रय आक्रान्त (71)

[During late summer], outside heat and internal cold (inside the body) gives rise to diseases caused by three, [viz., *rluṅ or vāyu, mkhris pa* or *pitta* and *bad kan* or *kapha*].

Regimens

Rluṅ nad bsal phyir lus mñe snum bsku sman chu bskol bas bkru //
वायु रोग प्रशम हेतु शरीर अभ्यंग स्निग्ध लेप भेषज जल शृत स्नान (72)

[During late summer] one should resort to oil massage, unctuous anointment and bath with medicine-boiled-water for the alleviation of *rluṅ* (*vāyu*).

Rluṅ nad sel ṅes[55] til mar mas btaṅ[56] dugs daṅ lums kyaṅ bya //
वायु रोग प्रशम निश्चय तिल तैल अनुवासन स्वेदन अवगाह कर्तव्य (73)

[During late summer] one should take medicated enema (*anuvāsana*) prepared of sessame oil and resort to fomentation through hot bath (*avagāha sveda*) in order to ensure alleviation of diseases caused by *rluṅ* (*vāyu*).

Food

Zas kyaṅ ha caṅ tsha min mṅar skyur med par raṅ par sbyar //
भोजन अधिक अनुष्ण मधुर अम्ल अप्राप्त यथायोग्य मिश्रित (74)

[During late summer], one should take more of food which are not hot and which are sweet and sour. If such food is not available then food should be mixed with appropriate ingredients.

57
Pho ba drod skyed bag daṅ mar tshil sbraṅ rtsi bar 'ga' bza' //
आमाशय उष्ण उत्पादन अन्न घृत वसा मधु अन्तरान्तरा भोजन (75)

[During late summer], one should eat food, butter, fat and honey at intervals with a view to promote digestive fire.

58
Yos daṅ 'bras chan mar khus blugs daṅ zan dron śa dag bza' //
भृष्टयव भृष्टशालि नवनीत मिश्रित शक्तु मांस भोजन 76)

[During late summer], one should take fried barley & fried rice added with melted butter, roasted corn flour and meat.

Drinks

59
Chaṅ yaṅ cuṅ zad btuṅ ste chu daṅ chu grog spaṅ bar bya //
मद्य अल्प पान जल नदीजल त्याग कर्तव्य (77)

[During late summer], one should drink less of alcohol and avoid drinking water [specially] river-water.

Other regimens

Rlan la mi 'dug mi 'gro lus la char pas gśer mi bya //
आर्द्र न निवास न गमन शरीर वर्षा सिक्त न कर्तव्य (78)

[During late summer], one should not stay in or go to a humid place, and during rains one should not get drenched.

Stobs dan drag śul nal źin dub par gyur pa'i bag dan yan //
साहस अतिव्यायाम श्रम मन्द आचरण अन्न लघु (79)

[During late summer], exhibition of strength, violent exercise and fatigue should be resorted to only moderately and one should take light food.

Ñin mtshan mi bde ñin par mi log ñal po brtun byed span //
दिवा रात्रि न सुख दिवा न निद्रा व्यवाय अतिक्लान्त त्याग (80)

[During late summer], one does not feel happy both during the day and night. He should not sleep and perform sexual intercourse during the day time and he should avoid excessively tiring efforts.

60
Gnas kyan rlan med rlun mi ldan la bsil bar stan gdin 'dug //
रहित
निवास आद्र रहित वायु (न प्रकोप) शीतल आस्तरण स्थान (81)

[During late summer], one should stay in a house free from humidity and (excessive) wind. If one feels cold then carpets should be spread [on the floor of the house].

REGIMENS FOR *STON* (AUTUMN)

Ston zla gñis ni mkhris pa skye ba'i dus yin nad ldaṅ bas //
शरत् मास द्वय पित्त जनन काल रोग उत्पन्न (82)

The two months of autumn causes aggravation of *mkhris pa* (*pitta*) as a result of which diseases are caused.

Bsil mṅar bkru sman gtaṅ źiṅ gtar kas khrag kyaṅ ci ran dbyuṅ //
शीतल मधुर विरेचन सेवन शिराव्यध रक्त यथायोग्य निर्हरण (83)

[During autumn] one should use cooling and sweet things, resort to purgation therapy and blood-letting therapy by venesection in appropriate manner.

Medicines

Kha źiṅ mṅar la bsil ba'i sman yaṅ rtag tu bza' bar bya //
तिक्त मधुर शीतल औषध लघु सदा भोजन कर्तव्य (84)

[During autumn] one should always use bitter, sweet, cooling and light medicines and food.

Water

Dus 'di'i chu ni dug med gtsaṅ daṅ bkrus śiṅ 'thuṅs na phan //
काल एतत् जल निर्विष निर्मल स्नान पान हितकर (85)

[During autumn] water is free from poisons and clean; therefore use of water during this season for bath and drink is beneficial.

Diet

Zas kyaṅ 'bras nas sran ma sbraṅ rtsi kha ra śa la sogs //
भोजन शालि यव शिम्बीधान्य मधु शर्करा मांस इत्यादि (86)

[During autumn] one should take rice, barley, pulses, honey, sugar, meat, etc., as food.

Drinks

Mṅar źiṅ kha la yaṅ ba mar sar o'ma bza' źiṅ btuṅ //
मधुर तिक्त लघु घृत दुग्ध भोजन पान (87)

[During autumn], one should take ingredients which are sweet, bitter and light [including] ghee and milk as food and drink.

Alcoholic drinks

Chaṅ lci drag po'i ro yod mi btuṅ ra ror mi bya ste //
मद्य गुरू तीक्ष्ण स्वादिष्ट न पान मत्तता न कर्तव्य (88)

[During autumn] one should not drink alcohol which is heavy, sharp and delicilous, and one should not get intoxicated by taking alcoholic drinks.

Tshil daṅ til mar mi bza' zil par mi 'gro 'dug mi bya //
मेदस् तिल तैल न भोजन तुषार न गमन निवास न कर्तव्य (89)

[During autumn], one should not eat fat and sessame oil and one should not walk or stay on forst.

Tsha ba'i zas daṅ yul yaṅ zla grogs yid du o'ṅ ba bsten //
उष्ण अन्न देश चन्द्र मित्र मनोरम उपभोग (90)

[During autumn] one should take hot food, stay in a warm place and enjoy moon, friend and such other pleasing things.

Chu 'jam tsam gyis lus bkru gos kyan dri ma med pa bgo //
उष्णोदक किंचित् शरीर स्नान वसन निर्मल परिधान (91)

[During autumn] one should take bath in small quantity of lukewarm water and wear clean cloth.

61 62 63 64
Rgyan dan dri źim lus la gdags śin ñin mtshan mi bde ste //
अलंकार सुगन्ध शरीर परिधान दिवा रात्र मनुष्य सुखी (92)

[During autumn] one should wear ornaments and apply scents over the body. As such, the person should spend day and night happily.

65
Gnas kyan dro min bser bus mi phog bsil bag can la 'dug //
आवास अनुष्ण निवात शीतल स्त्री सह वास (93)

[During autumn] one should stay in a place which is neither hot nor windy and one should live with conserts having cooling nature.

REGIMENS FOR *DGUN STOD* AND *DGUN SMAD* (EARLY AND LATE WINTERS)

66

Dgun stod dgun smad zla bźi phyi graṅ naṅ tsha bad kan gsog //
हेमन्त शिशिर मास चत्वार वाह्य शीतल अन्तः उष्ण कफ संचय (94)

During the four months of *dgun stood* (*hemanta* = early winter) and *dgun smad* (*śiśira* = late winter) out side it is cold and inside the body, it is hot. During this period *kapha* gets accumulated.

67 68

Gos dror bgo źiṅ rlan daṅ lhags la bag bya ñi ma'ṅ sdod //
वस्त्र उष्ण परिधान आर्द्र आगमन भोजन कर्तव्य दिवा अपि काम (95)

[During winter season], one should wear warm cloth, at the advent of humidity, one should eat and one should satisfy sexual desire even during the day time.

Food

69

Zas kyaṅ śa tshon rus khu mar tshil snum bag 'graṅs par bza' //
अन्न मांस मेदस्वी अस्थि रस धृत वसा स्निग्ध भोजन उदरपूर्ण भोजन (96)

[During early and late winter seasons] one should take bellyful of food mixed with meat of fatty animals, bone-soup, ghee, fat and oil.

Mṅar skyur lan tshwa drod bag cher bza' gsar tog 'bru dag bza' //
मधुर अम्ल लवण उष्ण भोजन अधिक भोजन नव धान्य भोजन (97)

[During early and late winter seasons] one should eat more of sweet, sour, saline and hot food in large quantities. One [can also] use freshly harvested corns.

Drink and regimons

Ran par sna tshogs chan btuṅ ṅal ba'i las dag byas kyaṅ sla //
सामान्य विविध मद्य पान व्यायाम कर्तव्य सुकर (98)

[During early and late winter seasons] one should drink different types of alcohal in moderate quantity and perform exercise as well as physical work.

70
Rtsol bcag lus sbyaṅ skabs skabs mgo lus til mar bsku ziṅ mñe //
सामान्य कर्म देह शोधन कदा कदा शिर शरीर तिल तैल लेप अभ्यंग (99)

[During early and late winter seasons,] one should perform normal work, cleanse the body [by purgation therapy] and occasionally (frequently) apply sessame oil over the head and body, and perform massage.

Bath

De rjes skyu ru ra la sogs pa sman bskol chus kyaṅ bkru //
तदनन्तर आमलकी इत्यादि औषध शृत जल स्नान (100)

[During early and late winter seasons,] one should thereafter [after oil massage] take bath in water boiled with medicines like *āmalakī* (*Emblica officinalis*), etc.

House and seat

Gnas kyaṅ bsro khaṅ dron por me daṅ stan stug ldan par 'dug //
गृह उष्ण गृह उष्ण अग्नि आसन स्थुल युक्त निवास (101)

[During early and late winter seasons,] one should stay in a hot house, near fire and sit over a thick [comfortably warm] seat.

Prohibitions for different seasons

Dbyar stod tsha dus dbyar smad rluṅ dus bkru sman mi gtaṅ ste //
ग्रीष्म उष्ण काल प्रावृट्‌ वायु काल विरेचन न सेवन (102)

First part of summer is hot and in the later part of summer *rluṅ (vāyu)* gets aggravated [Therefore, during these two seasons] purgation therapy should not be administered.

71

Dgun stod dgun smad graṅ daṅ rgas la skyug sman gtar ga spaṅ //
हेमन्त शिशिर शीत वृद्ध वमन शिराव्यध त्याग (103)

Early and later parts of winter are cold. During these seasons and to old persons, emetic theraphy and venesection should not be administered.

Dgun gnis dbyar stod lums dugs mi bya nad kyis gzir kyaṅ sla //
शीतकाल द्वय ग्रीष्म अवगाह स्वेदन न कर्तव्य व्याधि आक्रान्त परन्तु कर्तव्य (104)

During both the early and late winter seasons and during the summer season, one should not take medicated bath and fomentation therapies. If, however, a person is afflicted with diseases, these therapies may be administered to him.

De ltar yin yaṅ lus daṅ nad du gar mthun ba rtsam par bya //
तथाविध यत्रयत्र शरीर व्याधि उपयुक्त दृष्ट कर्तव्य (105)

In the same way, what so ever therapy is considered wholesome to the body and to the disease can be administered.

CONDUCT FOR POSITIVE HEALTH (PRESERVATION AND PROMOTION)

Rluṅ mkhris bad kan gsum daṅ 'phrod pas 'tsho ba'i mdo brjod nas //
वायु पित कफ त्रय हित आयु नियम निर्गदित (106)

Rules for the promotion of longevity are described above keeping in view the wholesome things for the three (elements); viz, *rluṅ* (*vāyu*), *mkhris pa* (*pitta*) and *bad kan (kapha)*.

Bag byed spyod lam can dag raṅ du 'tsho phyir yaṅ bstan pa //
संक्षेप चर्या आत्मन् आयु हेतु उपदिष्ट (107)

[Now], the conducts [which are useful for the promotion] of longevity of the person are being described.

Med smra cir yaṅ chos daṅ rigs pa gźan dag gsum la 'dzom //
विपरित भाषण सदा धर्म विद्या अपर त्रय त्याग (108)

Negative speaking and speaking out [secrets of] others religion as well as knowledge, these three should always be avoided.

72 73
Sṅar byas naṅ nub bsam źiṅ skyor dor phyiṅ chad bag cher bya //
पूर्व कृत पश्चात् चिन्तन पुनः त्याग अग्रे पश्चाताप अल्पाधिक कर्तव्य (109)

One should think his [misdeeds] of the past and should not repeat them. He should repent for these misdeeds appropriately in future.

Byed pa gaṅ la rdul med raṅ ñam med ciṅ 'dod chen spaṅ //
कार्य किंचित् धूलि न आत्म भय न काम अधिक त्याग (110)

While performing what so over work one should not throw-dust, one should not have fear-complex and one should not have sex desires in excess.

74 75 76
Ṅa rgyal loṅs sphyod spyi brtol che min śed dman khum mi bya //
अहंकार काम निर्लज्ज अधिक न कथन नीच अश्लील न कर्तव्य (111)

One should not be egoistic, should not be sexy and should not indulge in shameless talk. One should avoid mean and vulgar activities.

77 78
Sdig grogs spaṅ źin dge bśes bsten te gtoṅ smos dge bcu spyad //
पापी मित्र त्याग कल्याण मित्र सेवन शुभदान कथन मंगल दश सेवन (112)

One should shun friendship with sinful persons, attend to auspicious friends, speak of auspicious charity and rejoice ten auspicious things.

Following are the ten auspicious things according to Buddhism :

(A) Of body
(1) *Srog mi gcod pa* (*ahiṁsā* = nonviolence)
(2) *Ma byin par mi lan pa* (*asteya* = non-stealing)
(3) *Tshaṅs par spyod pa* (*nirmala* caritra = to observe moral purity)

(B) Of speech
(4) *Bden par smra pa* (*satya bhāṣaṇa* = to speak truth)
(5) *Thsig 'jam por smra pa* (*vinaya bhāṣaṇa* = to speak politely)
(6) *Ṅag mi 'chal pa* (*pratijña pālana* = not to break promise)
(7) *Phra pa mi byed pa* (*parapakathana tyāga* = not to speak slander)

(C) Of mind
(8) *Gźan gyi nor la ham pa mi byed pa* (*para dravya alobhna* = not to covet for others property)
(9) *Gźan la gnod pa'i sems mi bskyed pa* (*para dveṣa tyāga* = not to think ill of others)
(10) *Yaṅ dag pa'i lta ba* (*samyak śāśana pālana* = to respect the purest doctrine)

Gsoṅ des tshul chags gźan la gnod min mi la byams par bya //
पूर्वाभिभाषी भद्र शील स्नेह अपर पीडा न मनुष्य मैत्री कर्तव्य (113)

One should wish others before he is wished, exhibit noble conduct and love for others. One should not harm any body and should have friendship with others.

79 80
Lha daṅ rgyal por ñer bsam luṅ mñan yid daṅ mthun par sgrub //
देव राजा यथायोग्य भावना आदेश श्रवण मनस् अनुकूल साधन (114)

One should have appropriate respect for God and King, should respectfully hear their instructions and should perform such action as are conducive to them (God and King).

81
Rgyal po'i sras daṅ rma ni chuṅ yaṅ mi brñas bag cher bya //
राजा कुमार सौन्दर्य अल्प न अवमानना यथायोग्य कर्तव्य (115)

One should not show disrespect to the King's son even if he is unsuitable for the position (less beautiful). One should behave with such persons appropriately.

Spyod lam sgyu mas mi bslu bka' khrims yul chos bsruṅ //
चर्या विकार न अपचिन्तन राजनियम देश धर्म रक्षण (116)

One should not get deceived by perversion of conduct and one should follow (protect) the rules of the state, country and religion.

This line has only eleven words. Perhaps two words are mising and that has made its meaning clumsy.

82 83
Gźan gyi dpyas skyon mi brjod rtog 'dod gtum chos 'gran mi bya //
अपर न्यूनता दोष न कथन तर्क इच्छा क्रोध धर्म प्रतिस्पर्धा न कर्तव्य (117)

One should not speak about short comings and fault of others. One should shun the desire to have argument, anger or competition with other's religion.

84

Dge sloṅ slob dpon pha ma'i goṅ du mi 'gro sri źu skyed //
भिक्षु आचार्य पिता माता सम्मुख न गमन सम्मान उत्पादन (118)

One should not move ahead of monks, preceptors , father and mother. One should act before them with respect.

85

Dge sbyoṅ draṅ sroṅ srog chags ya mtshan mñan gtod sbrul mi rtse //
श्रमण ऋषि प्राणी सिद्ध श्रवण प्रणिपात सर्प न क्रीड़ा (119)

One should hear respectfully and submit to ascetics, saints, living beings and mystics. One should not play or have affection for snakes.

Ma rtogs śiṅ chen mchod rten druṅ daṅ lam mdo phug stod daṅ //
न ज्ञात वृक्ष महान् चैत्य निकट चतुष्पथ गुफा शुन्यस्थान (120)

86

Sems can maṅ du bsad pa'i slo sa dur khrod ñal mi bya //
प्राणी अधिक वध मलत्याग भूमि श्मशान निद्रा न कर्तव्य (121)

One should not sleep in an unknown [place, under] a big tree, in the compound of a religious monument, in cross-roads, in a cave, in an empty house, in a place where animals are slaughtered, in a place used for the evacuation of stool and in a crematorium.

Gñan pa'i mtshod daṅ chu mig bzaṅ por mi bkru mi bśal te //
क्रूर ह्रद झर खरस्रोतस् न स्नान न प्रक्षालन (122)

One should not take bath or wash his body in a floaded lake or spring with strong current.

Rdo śiṅ dgon pa'i śiṅ chen mi bcad pha boṅ gźom mi bya //
पाषाण काष्ठ अरण्य महावृक्ष न कर्त्तन वृहत्पाषाण भंग न कर्त्तव्य (123)

One should not cut big trees in the forests of trees and stones and should not try to break big boulders.

87 88
Mchod rten rgyal mtshan ā rya'i grib ma ma ṇḍa la mi 'gom źin //
चैत्य ध्वज आचार्य छाया मण्डल न अतिक्रमण (124)

One should not walk over the shadow of religious monuments, [sacred] flags or preceptors. One also should not tread over the mystic and sacred circles [in religious places].

89 90
Mi ro gtor ma yas stegs ho ma khuṅ thal khuṅ bcag mi bya //
शव बलि वेदी होम कुण्ड भस्म कुण्ड भंग न कर्त्तव्य (125)

One should not break (scattar) a dead body, sacrificial offering, seat [of the gods & saints], place of sacrificial offerings and place of sacred ashes.

Nam mkha' ban bun ñi ma phyed daṅ dmar thag chad pa'i tshe //
आकाश खण्डित दिन अर्ध प्रत्यूष (सन्ध्या) समय (126)

91
Mi bza' mi btuṅ yi ge klog min ñal po las yaṅ spaṅ //
न भोजन न पान अक्षर पठन न मैथुन कर्म त्याग (127)

One should avoid taking food and drinks, study, and sexual intercourse when the sky appears broken, during midday and during dawn and dusk.

Ban bun in the text should better read *bun bun.*

Ñi ma la sogs o'd zer phra sdags mi riṅ riṅ mi blta //
सूर्य इत्यादि किरण तीक्षण न अतिकाल न दर्शन (128)

One should not look at the sharp rays of the sun, etc., for a long time.

Lha khaṅ sgor mi ñal te ri sna grog snar gnas mi bca' //
मंदिर परिधि न शयन पर्वत शिखर नदीतट विस्तार स्थान न निवास (129)

One should not sleep in the compound cf a temlple and should not reside [in a house] located at the top of a mountain or on the river-bank (ravine).

Ya mtshan śes drag mi bsten bud med ṅag mi mñan //
हास्य ज्ञान गरिमा न दर्शन स्त्री कथा न श्रवण (130)

One should not ridicule others and should not exhibit superiority of one's own knowledge. One should not be guided by the advice of women or one should not talk about women.

Bsten appearing in the text should better read *bstan*.

92

Bud med rgan la mi rgyo rtsal rgyos smra 'gros dub mi bya //
स्त्री वृद्धा न रमण साहस मैथुन भाषण गमन क्लान्त न कर्त्तव्य (131)

One should not indulge in sex with an old woman and one should not get fatigued by the exhibition of excessive strength, by sexual intercourse, by long & loud talks and by walking a long distance.

93

Gad mo che ziṅ riṅ du dgod daṅ ṅud mo drag po spaṅ //
हास्य उच्च अधिक काल परिहास क्रन्दन उच्चस्वर त्याग (132)

One should avoid loud laughing, playing jokes for a long time and crying in high pitch.

Rtag tu mi 'dug riṅ du mi 'gren ci nus ran par bcag //
सदा न उपवेशन अधिक काल न उत्थान यथा शक्ति उपयुक्त प्रदर्शन (133)

One should not sit and stand continuously for a long time and should exhibit his strength only according to his capacity [and not in excess].

NON-SUPPRESSION OF NATURAL URGES

Sbrig pa lud pa khu chu mchim snabs 'phyen[94] bśan gci g'yal[95] //
क्षवथु कास शुक्र अश्रु सिंघाणक वात पुरीष मूत्र जृम्भा (134)

Mi dgag ma bsgrus bkres skom nad gñid gnag min myur du bsal //
न रोध न प्रेरण क्षुधा तृषा रोग निद्रा रोध न शीघ्र उद्घाटन (135)

One should not suppress [the natural and manifested urges of] sneezing, coughing, ejaculation of semen, coming out of tears, excretion of the mucus from the nose, voiding flatus, stool and urine, yawning, hunger, morbid thirst and sleep. One also should not forcibly get these urges manifested. After their manifestation, these urges should be appropriately released quickly.

In ayurveda thirteen natural urges are described. These are (1) *mūtra* (urination), (2) *purīṣa* (voiding stool), (3) *retas* (ejaculating semen), (4) *vāta* (voiding flatus), (5) *chardi* (vomiting), (6) *kṣavathu* (sneezing), (7) *udgāra* (eructation) (*kāsa* or coughing according to *Vāgbhaṭa*), (8) *jṛmbhā* (yawning), (9) *kṣudhā* (hunger), (10) *pipāsā* (thirst), (11) *aśru* (tears), (12) *nidrā* (sleep) and *śrama svāsa* (urge for deep breathing because of exertion).

GENERAL CONDUCT FOR GOOD HEALTH

96 97
Ñal po skigs pa lud pa la sogs tshe lus mdzin mi gcu //
निद्रा हिक्का कास इत्यादि काल देह ग्रीवा न संकोचन (136)

One should not squeeze the body and the neck during sleep, attending to attacks of hiccup, cough, etc.

98
Glal na kha dgab sbrid pa smra tshe ha can kha mi bgrad //
जृम्भा मुख आवरण क्षवथु शब्द तीव्र अधिक मुख न अनावरण (137)

During yawning one should cover his mouth [with the hand], during sneezing one should not produce loud sound and one should not keep his mouth open.

Sen mo rin du mi bźag bregs te phan tshun brud mi bya //
नख अधिक काल न धारण कर्त्तन परस्पर घर्षण न कर्त्तव्य (138)

One should not keep nails [growing] for a long time. One should prune nails [regularly] and should not rub-nails with each other.

99 100
Mgo lus lag pas mi brdab mgo bo drag tu mi sprugs te //
शिरस् शरीर हस्त न पीडन शिरस् सशक्त न कम्पन (139)

One should not get the head and the body [forcibly] pressed by hands, and one should not shake the head violently.

Don med sa mi bri źin lag pa mi brdab mchu mi bri //
अर्थ रहीत भूमि न दारण हस्त न पीडन ओष्ठ न दारण (140)

One should not scratch the earth (ground) without any purpose; one should not [forcibly] press hands; and one should not scratch lips.

101 102 103 104
Mi nus bźin du lci mi gdags te mya nan mnan mi bya //
न शक्ति अनुसार गुरु न वहन दुःख रोध न कर्त्तव्य (141)

One should not lift (carry) heavy things [in excess of] one's strength and one should not suppress his sorrowful feelings.

105
Dpyid dan dbyar stod ston ni phyugs mar dus gźan til mar gyis //
वसन्त ग्रीष्म शरत् प्राणी वसा काल अन्य तिल तैल (142)

Rtag tu mgo dan rkan mthil bsku źin bar bar lus kyan bsku //
सदा सिरस् पाद तल अभ्यंग कदाकदा शरीर अभ्यंग (143)

In spring, summer and autumn seasons one should have the massage of the head and sole of the feet with animal fat. In other seasons, the massage should be performed with the help of sessame oil. At times, this massage should be performed for the entire body.

106 107
Ston dpyid ma yin dus gźan res 'ga' sna dan rna bar til mar blugs //
शरत् वसन्त अन्यत् काल अन्यत् कदाकदा नासा कर्ण तिल तैल पूरण (144)

In seasons, other than autumn and spring, one should at times pour sessame oil into the ears and nose.

Skyer pa'i kha nda stan zil dag gis bar bar mig kyan bku //
दार्वी खण्ड रसांजन कदाकदा चक्षु लेपन (अंजन) (145)

At times, one should apply the collyrium prepared of *dāru haridrā* (*Berberis aristata*) and *stan zil* (*rasāñjana* or antimony) in the eyes.

Rtag tu lus kyi byi dor bya źin sman snags rin chen gdags //
सदा देह शोधन कर्त्तव्य औषधि मंत्र मणि धारण (146)

Always one should keep the body clean and wear talishmans containing sacred drugs and incantations as well as gems and jewels.

108
Ser bu drag po mi ro'i dri dan dud pas phog mi bya //
शीतवात क्रूर शव गन्ध धूम्र सम्पर्क न कर्त्तव्य (147)

One should not come in contact with fierceful cold wind, smell of dead bodies and smoke.

109 110
Chu tshas mgo lus mi bkru bkru sman skyug sman gtan ba dan //
उष्णजल शिरस् शरीर न स्नान विरेचन औषधि वमन औषधि प्रयोग (148)

One should not wash the head and body with excessively hot water and should use purgative and emetic medicines (therapies)..

Cham pa ma źus btab ste mgo lus mi bkru snum mi bsku //
प्रतिश्याय अजीर्ण आक्रान्त शिरस् देह न स्नान तैल न अभ्यंग (149)

If there is attack of cold or indigestion, then one should not wash the head and the body and one should not apply oil over the head and the body.

111 112
Skya rens śar nas tsog pur 'dug ste de rin ci bya bsam //
प्रत्यूष उत्थान अनन्तर प्रांजलि आसन उपवेशन तद्द दिन किं कर्त्तव्य चिन्तन (150)

One should get up from the bed early in the morning, sit with folded hands (in the pose of prayer) and think of the task to be performed on that day.

113
Lans nas so śin bca' źin kha yi skyon bsal lag gdon bkru //
उत्थान अनन्तर दन्तकाष्ठ भक्षण मुख दोष दोष शोधन हस्त मुख प्रक्षालन (151)

After getting up from the bed, one should clean his mouth of dirt by chewing (brushing with) tooth-stick and then wash his face and hands.

De nas sman mchog a ru ra ni rtag zos bdud rtsi yin //
तदनन्तर औषधि श्रेष्ठ हरीतकी सदा भक्षण अमृत (152)

Thereafter, one should always eat *a ru ra* (*harītakī = Terminalia chebula*) which is the best among medicines and it works like ambrosia.

Lug gi mar min mar sar źun mar rgas sra tshe riṅ ste //
मेष वसा अलाभ नवनीत घृत वार्धक्य देहसंघात दीर्घायु (153)

One should take the fat of sheep, or in case of its nonavailability one should take butter and ghee for the prevention of aging process and for the promotion of compactness of the body as well as longevity.

'Di la sogs pa lus daṅ tshe la phan pa'i sman zos na //
तद्‌ इत्यादि शरीर आयु हित औषध भक्षण (154)

The above mentioned medicines and such other medicines as are beneficial for the body and life should be taken.

114

Byug pa rgyan daṅ gos kyis śin du mdzes byas lha yaṅ mchod //
धारण अलंकार वस्त्र अति सुन्दर परिधान देव प्रार्थना (155)

After wearing ornaments and beautiful cloth one should offer prayer to the gods.

115

De nas sri źu'i gnas daṅ 'khor la sñan brjod 'dzum bstan nas //
तदनन्तर पूजास्थान (मित्र) परिवार श्रवण कथन स्मित दर्शन (156)

Thereafter, one should politely and smilingly talk to and hear from respected friends and family members.

116
Rje dpon las daṅ bdag gźan don la naṅ tan brtson 'grus skyed //
गुरु कार्य आत्मन् अपर अर्थ उद्यम प्रयत्न उत्साह जनन (157)

One should do service to preceptor and strive to perform duties for himself and for others which gives rise to enthusiasm.

117 118
Dus bźir dro bab ran par zas bza' ṅoms par skom 'thuṅ ste //
काल तत्वारः भोजन ग्रहण सम्यक् अन्न भक्षण संतोष तृष्णा पान (158)

One should eat food in moderate quantity four times per day and after being satisfied with the food, he should drink for the alleviation of thirst.

Thug pa khu tshan la sogs snum lci drod kun sṅar bza' źiṅ //
यूष रस उष्ण इत्यादि स्निग्ध गुरु अग्निदीपन पूर्व भोजन (159)

Prior to taking meals, one should take vegetable soup, hot meat soup, etc., which are unctuous, heavy and promoter of digestion.

119 120
'Bras la sogs pa bsil yaṅ phyis bza' 'phrad med phye ma 'gam //
शालि अन्न इत्यादि शीत लघु अनन्तर भक्षण अमिश्रित शक्तु न भक्षण(160)

[After the intake of soup], one should take rice, etc., which are cooling and light. One should not take roasted corn flour without adding [spices].

Bab chol ha caṅ 'graṅs par bza' min myos par chaṅ mi btuṅ //
शीघ्र अधिक उदरपूर्ण भक्षण न तीव्र (मादक) मद्य न पान (161)

One should not take food in haste, in more quantity and to the full of one's stomach-capacity. One should not drink strong (intoxicating) alcohol.

'Bras kyis 'grans rjes phye zan mi bza' drod rjes skom mi btun //
शालि अन्न उदरपूर्ण अनन्तर शक्तु भोजन न भक्षण उष्ण अनन्तर तृष्णा न पान(162)

One should not eat roasted corn-flour after taking bellyful of rice, and he should not drink if he feels thirsty after taking hot food.

121 122 123
Skyo ma ran par 'thuns na lus brta nan na rgan la bsod //
यवागू यथाकाल पान देह विस्तार अन्तः वृद्ध उत्तम (163)

If one drinks gruel in appropriate time, then it gets expanded inside [the stomach]. It is useful for old persons.

124 125
Bro drug gan yan gcig la cher zos nad ldan par sbyar //
रस षड् यत्किंचित् एक अधिक भक्षण रोग कारक मिश्रण (164)

Diseases are caused by the intake of ingredients having only one of tastes in excess. Therefore, ingredients having different tastes should be appropriately mixed together and taken.

'Grans pa'i rjes la ñal po ban stobs rta rgyug la sogs span //
उदरपूर्ण (भोजन) अनन्तर शयन धावन श्रम अश्वारोहण इत्यादि त्याग (165)

After the intake of bellyful of food one should avoid sleep, running, hard work, horse-riding, etc.

126
Śiṅ tog ldam ldum maṅ na nad ldaṅ ba mos phog pa gnod //
फल निन्द्य अधिक रोग उत्पन्न ओषयुक्त अहितकर (166)

Fruits are not useful. If used in excess, they cause diseases. When exposed to dew-drops, these are harmful for the stomach.

127 128
Dbyar zla 'briṅ po'i tshes la ldam ldum bza' drag nad du 'gyur //
ज्येष्ठ मास मध्यम काल निन्द्य भक्षण तीव्र रोग जनन (167)

The month of *dbyar* (*jyeṣṭha* = Aprīl-May) is of mediocre nature and during this month if bad food is taken in excess, then it gives rise to serious diseases.

Nad can lums kyis draṅs te mgyogs na nad ldaṅ skran du o'ṅ //
रोगी अवगाह शीर्ण शीघ्र रोग संक्रमण गुल्म आगमन (168)

If the patient becomes weak because of hot medicated bath, then he quickly falls victims to diseases like *skran* (*gulma* = phantom tumour).

MUTUALLY CONTRADICTORY FOOD AND DRINKS

Mchin pa g'yer ma spaṅs te zos na cuṅ zad sñiṅ la gnod //
यकृत वन्य मरिच त्याग भोजन अल्प हृदय अहितकर (169)

One should not eat liver with wild capsicum (*gyer ma = vanya marica*). If it is to be eaten, then it should be taken only in small quantity because it is harmful for the heart.

Zas mchog sbraṅ rtsi mar ñiṅ cha mñam zos na dug bźin gnod //
भोजन उत्तम मधु घृत पुराण भाग सम भक्षण विष वत् अहितकर (170)

Honey and old ghee, these two are the best among the food ingredients. But if taken in equal quantities, these work like poison, and therefore, harmful.

129

Mi mñam che chuṅ byas kyaṅ zos rjes chaṅ chu 'thuṅs na gnod //
न सम अधिक अल्प कृत भक्षण अनन्तर मद्य मण्ड पान अहितकर (171)

[Honey and old ghee] should be taken in unequal quantities, one in less and the other in more quantity. Even after taking these ingredients in unequal quantities, if one takes *chaṅ chu* (*sura maṇḍa* = upper part of aicohol) then it is harmful.

130

Ma laṅs źo daṅ laṅs ma thag gi źo dron nad kun sloṅ //
तरुण दधि पक्व न गत दधि उष्ण रोग सर्व उत्पन्न (172)

Intake of immature (not formented) curd or the curd which is not fully formented (immediately after formentation) gives rise to all heating diseases.

131
Chu bya dbyar spaṅ ldum mchog ke'u ni dbyar zla 'briṅ po'i sman //
जलकुक्कुट ग्रीष्म त्याग शाक श्रेष्ठ गृंजनक ज्येष्ठ औषधि (173)

One should give up taking meat of water fowl in the summer. *Ke'u* (*gṛñjanaka* = carrot) is the best among vegetables. It is the medicine of the middle of the summer months (*jyeṣṭha* or April-May; it works as a preventive medicine).

132 133
Sman 'thuṅs śa ba'i śa gnod ga gon źo 'drer rims su 'gyur //
औषध पान मृग मांस अहितकर कर्कोटी दधि मिश्रण संक्रामकरोग उत्पन्न (174)

Eating the meat of large stag after drinking medicinal decoctions is bad. Intake of cucumber with curd produces diseases.

Brtsoṅ bsregs sbraṅ rtsir mi 'phrod lhan cig zos na 'chi bar 'gyur //
पलाण्डु दग्ध मधु न हित एकत्र भक्षण मृत्यु प्राप्ति (175)

Intake of burnt onion with honey is unwholesome. Taking this combined food even once causes death.

Ke'u a'm gnag śa lhan cig zos na skran du 'gyur //
गृंजनक चर्म्मरी मांस एकत्र भक्षण गुल्म प्राप्ति (176)

Intake of *ke'u* (*gṛñjanaka* = carrot) along with the meat of yak (black - cattle) together, produces *kran* (*gulma* = phantom tumour)

134 135
Dgun stod rgya g'yer zos na sñiṅ ni drags na mig kyaṅ mdoṅs //
हेमन्त हरिण वन्यमरिच भक्षण हृदय अतिमात्र चक्षु आन्ध्य (177)

Intake of deer-meat with *g'yer* (*vana marica* = wild capsicum) in early winter is harmful for the heart. If taken in excess, it causes blindness of the eyes.

Mar tshil zos dan mi 'phrod lha ba bza' drags na so 'byun //
नवनीत वसा भक्षण न सात्म्य पूति भक्षण अतिमात्र सुख उत्पन्न (178)

Intake of butter along with fat is unwholesome. Intake of these items after preservation for a long time and in large quantity endows happiness.

136

Bra bo man du zos na rlun dan lus g'ya' ste //
फाफर अधिक भक्षण वायु शरीर कण्डू (179)

Intake of buck-wheat in excess aggravates *rluṅ* (*vāyu*) and causes itching in the body.

This line of the text has only eleven words. Two words appear to have been omitted through over sight during calligraphy.

137

Nub mo chu 'thun chan gnon la phug rñid dan śa skam span //
सांय जल पान मद्य पान मूलक पुराण (शीर्ण) मांस शुष्क त्याग (180)

In the evening one should avoid taking water, alcohol, over-matured radish and dry meat.

Ña dan kha tsha mar tshil mi 'phrod snod kyan gcig mi bya //
मत्स्य तिक्त कटु नवनीत वसा न सात्म्य भाण्ड एक न कर्त्तव्य (181)

Intake of bitter and pungent [spices] along with fish is unwholesome. Intake of butter and animal fat together is unwholesome. One should not cook all these ingredients in one vessel.

Ña dan o'ma lhan cig man zos nan na zer ma gnod //
मत्स्य दुग्ध एकत्र अधिक भक्षण आभ्यन्तर (?) अहितकर (182)

Intake of fish and milk together in excess quantity produce harmful effect inside the body inasmuch as it causes leprosy.

Zer ma (lit. a drop) in the above text appears to be an error. It should better read *mdze* meaning leprosy. Translation is made accordingly.

Śiṅ tog chaṅ la sogs te skyur daṅ śaṅ tshe la phug sloṅ //
फल मद्य इत्यादि अम्ल (?) मूलक आर्द्र (183)

138
Yuṅs rñiṅ 'di rnams gaṅ yaṅ o'mar 'phrod min maṅ zos gnod //
सर्षप पुराण एते यत्किंचित् दुग्ध सात्म्य न अधिक भक्षण अहितकर (184)

Intake of sour things like fruits, alochol, etc., *śaṅ tshe* (?), green radish and old mustard, any of these ingredients, along with milk is not wholesome. Taking such combined food in large quantity is harmful.

139
O' tshan 'thuṅs rjes chu grog 'thuṅs daṅ rgya sran nag po gnod //
दुग्ध उष्ण पान अनन्तर जल शीतल पान शमीधान्य कृष्ण अहितकर (185)

Intake of black-gram after taking hot milk or cold water (spring water) is harmful.

140
Zla ba sbyaṅ kis zin tshe zan zos so na śu ba 'byuṅ //
चन्द्र ग्रहण काल अन्न भक्षण दन्तविद्रधि जात (186)

Intake of food during lunar eclipse gives rise to dental tumour(abcess).

Gnag śa rta śa lhan cig zos na lus la g'yan pa o'ṅ //
चर्म्मरी मांस अश्व मांस एकत्र भक्षण शरीर कण्डू जात (187)

Intake of meat of yak and horse together gives rise to iches in the body.

Gnag śa phag śa lhan cig zos na lto yi srin bur 'gyur //
चर्म्मरी मासं शूकर मांस एकत्र भक्षण उदर कृमि जात (188)

Intake of the meat of yak and pig together produces warms in the stomach.

Ña daṅ khyim bya'i śa gñis lhan cig zos na skran du 'gyur //
मत्स्य गृह कुक्कुट मांस द्वय एकत्र भक्षण गुल्म जात (189)

Intake of fish and chicken together produces *skran* (*gulma* = phantom tumour).

Khyim bya'i sgo ṅa'i spri daṅ sgog skya zos na dbug mi bde //
गृह कुक्कुट अण्ड पीतभाग लशुन भक्षण श्वास (190)

Intake of the yalk of the egg of domesticated fowl together with (white) garlic produces asthma.

141

Khyim bya'i śa daṅ ri boṅ śa gñis lhan cig zos na cuṅ zad 'khru //
गृह कुक्कुट मांस शशक मांस द्वय एकत्र भक्षण अल्प ग्रहण अतिसार (191)

Intake of the meat of domestic fowl and rabbit together, even in small quantity, produces diarrhoea.

Śa mo yuṅs mar naṅ du brdos pa zos na lus la gnod //
छत्रक सर्षप तैल भर्जित भक्षण देह अहितकर (192)

Intake of mushrooms fried with mustard oil is harmful for the body.

142

Ma nu'i sa bon ka tsam tsi daṅ sbraṅ rtsir 'phrod ma yin //
पुष्कर बीज वन्यमुद्ग जूर्णाह्व मधु सात्म्य न (193)

Intake of the seeds of *ma nu* (*puṣkara* = *Inula racemosa*) along with wild oat, millet and honey is not wholeshome.

La phug bu ram mi 'phrod źo daṅ bya gag śar mi 'phrod //
मूलक गुड न सात्म्य दधि वक मांस न सात्म्य (194)

Radish and jaggery, mixed together, are not wholesome. Similarly, meat of crane mixed with curd is unwholesome.

De ltaṅ 'phrod zas goms daṅ rtag tu chags pa daṅ //
तथा सात्म्य अन्न अभ्यास सदा अनुरक्त (195)

Laṅ tsho 'ju slas zos daṅ ñuṅ na gnod pa med daṅ bsre //
यौवन सुपाच्य अन्न अल्प अहित न मिश्रण (196)

'Phrod pa'i zas zos phyi dro'i las byas nam sros bde bar ñal //
सात्म्य अन्न भक्षण अपराह्ण कर्म कर्त्तव्य रात्रि सुख स्वप्न (197)

De ltar nan tan bag byas mi tshe tshad bźin 'tsho des pas //
तथा उद्यम भोजन कर्त्तव्य मनुष्य आयुस् मान तथा जीवन पेशल (198)

Habitual intake of wholesome food, constant love [for others], youthful age, intake of easily digestible food, avoiding even small quantity of harmful food, intake of food mixed with wholesome ingredients, work in the afternoon, good sleep at night, professional duty and [regular] intake of food prolong the span of life and keep a person happy.

SPAN OF LIFE - DUTIES IN DIFFERENT STAGES

143 144

Skyes nas lo bcu'i bar du sma mi dbab cin ran dgar gźag //
जन्म वर्ष दश काल नम्र नर प्रवेश स्वयं सुख स्थित (199)

From birth uptill ten years of age, a person remains humble and self-contented.

145

De nas ñi śu lon te lo bcur bslab dan brtsal bar bya //
तदनन्तर विशंति प्रवेश वर्ष दश शिक्षा कर्त्तव्य कर्म कर्त्तव्य (200)

Thereafter, for ten years i.e. upto the time when he enters twentieth year of age, he should get education and prform his [professional] duties.

146

De nas lṅa bcu lṅa lon sum cu rtsa lṅa khyud 'khor du //
तदनन्तर पंचपंचाशत् प्रवेश पंचत्रिंश पूजन परिवार (201)

Lons spyod grags pa'i yul srid gtam byas nas //
भोग यश देश आरोह प्रवचन करण (202)

For thirty five years thereafter, *i.e.* upto the arrival of the age of fifty five, a person should perform religious duties, enjoy pleasures of family life, attain fame, visit various countries and deliver [religious]speeches.

Lṅa bcu lṅa lon phyin chad chos lam yum gyi ched bsgrub phyir //
पंचपंचाशत् प्रवेश उपरान्त सन्यास धर्म मार्ग मातृ निमित्त साधन हेतु (203)

Dge la btson bskyed thos rig goms byed lus sems ci bder gnas //
कल्याण कर्म उत्पन्न श्रवण ज्ञान अभ्यास करण देह मनस किं सुख स्थान (204)
(विद्या)

De ltar sus nus mi lus thob pa'i don yod skyid cin dge //
तथा भद्र शक्ति नर देह प्राप्ति अर्थ अस्ति सुख कल्याण (205)

After fifty five years of age, one should be free (live like on ascetic) to serve the mother religion, i.e engage himself in religious practices, to resort to auspicious activities, to hear and learn religions scriptures, to practice the commandments in one's own life, and to realise the factors responsible for happiness of the body as well as the mind. Because of these, a person aquires the power of auspiciousness and benedictory objects of obtaining [human] body which gives rise to [eternal] happiness.

Colophon

Slob dpon 'phags pa Klu-sgrub-sñiṅ pos sman rnams la brdzaṅs pa //
आचार्य आर्य नागार्जुन-हृदय वैद्य निगदित (206)

Sman 'tsho-ba'i mdo tshigs su bcad pa rdzogs so //
वैद्य जीव सूत्र पद्य रचित समाप्त (207)

Thus, ends the Vaidya Jīva Sūtra composed in verses by preceptor Ārya Nāgārjuna Hṛdaya for the [benefit of] physicians.

FOOT NOTES

(1) Sman 'tsho ba'i mdo Klu-sgrub-kyis mdzad pa bźugs (N & P); bźug pa (D); bźugs so (J)
(2) bcal (N & P)
(3) bsdus (N & P)
(4) brtags (N & P)
(5) spyad (N & P)
(6) blta (N & P)
(7) sogs (D & J)
(8) sogs (D & J)
(9) sogs (D & J)
(10) bro (D & J)
(11) bskyed (N & P)
(12) mu ga (N & P)
(13) sbyaṅ rtsi (J)
(14) sñiṅ (P)
(15) bskyed (N & P)
(16) bskyed (N)
(17) bskyed (N)
(18) bskyed (N)
(19) gsum pa (D & J)
(20) maṅs (N & P)
(21) skye (D & J)
(22) tshwa (P)
(23) las (D & J)
(24) tsha (N)
(25) rim pa (N)
(26) tshwa (P)
(27) mar (D & J)
(28) bźin (N)
(29) tsha (N)
(30) tshwa (P)
(31) mṅar (N & P)
(32) gsum ga (P)
(33) bskyed (N & P)
(34) Not available in P
(35) 'phros (P)
(36) bskyod (N & P)
(37) rga (N & P)
(38) ñiṅ (P); ñid (D & J)
(39) btud (P)
(40) rlu (P)
(41) śiṅ (P)
(42) las (D, N & P)
(43) 'jug (J)
(44) ma (D)
(45) graṅs (N & P)
(46) lan tsha (D)
(47) yogs (N & P)
(48) rñan (N)
(49) chad (N & P)
(50) bser (N & P)
(51) sogs (D & J)
(52) ciṅ (N & P)
(53) gaṅ (N)
(54) g'yo (N & P)
(55) des (D)
(56) gtoṅ (D & J)
(57) bskyed (N)
(58) khu blug (N & P)
(59) 'grog (P), 'grogs (N)
(60) btiṅ (D & J)
(61) gṅags (N & P)
(62) ñi (N & P)
(63) tshan (N & P)

(64) lde (N & P)
(65) ser (D & J)
(66) sogs (D & J)
(67) pa (C, P & J)
(68) 'di (D); lda (N); sdo (P); 'de (J)
(69) tshig (N & P)
(70) rtsel (D); rtsal (N & P)
(71) gtar ka (P)
(72) skyen (N)
(73) chag (N,P,D & J)
(74) laṅ tshos (D & J)
(75) śes (D & J)
(76) źus (N & P)
(77) gśes (P)
(78) spaṅ (N)
(79) mñam (N & P)
(80) bsgrub (P)
(81) bsñas (P)
(82) gyis spyas (N & P)
(83) rtogs (P), grtogs (N)
(84) bskyed (N)
(85) brtse (N & P)
(86) bsad pa (N & P)
(87) a rag'i (D & J)
(88) 'goṅ (D & J)
(89) stags (D & J), btags (N&P)
(90) gral (p)
(91) daṅ yaṅ (D & J); daṅ spaṅ (N & P)
(92) rgyo (N & P)
(93) rgod (P)
(94) phyen (N & P)
(95) dbyal; dbyal (gyal) (J)
(96) skegs (P); skyigs bu (J)
(97) tshi (N)
(98) me (N & P)
(99) la (N & P)
(100) sprug (N & P)
(101) nu (N & P)
(102) ci (D)
(103) 'dags (N & P)
(104) gnan (D)
(105) bźin (D, P & J)
(106) dus gźan not available in (P & N)
(107) blug (N)
(108) bser (N & P)
(109) btaṅ (N)
(110) la (P)
(111) reṅ (N)
(112) por (N & P)
(113) gsal (P)
(114) tu (N)
(115) srid (N)
(116) bskyed (N & P)
(117) ba (P)
(118) btuṅ (N & P)
(119) phrad (N & P)
(120) bkam (P)
(121) rta (N & P)
(122) rga naṅ (P)
(123) gsod (N & P)
(124) ro (N & P)
(125) zod naṅ (P)
(126) maṅs (N & P)
(127) 'briṅ po (N)
(128) drags (N & P)
(129) du (D & J)
(130) kloṅ (P)
(131) ki lun (N & P)
(132) źor (N & P)
(133) 'dres (N & P)
(134) na (P)
(135) lčoṅ (N & P)
(136) do (p)
(137) sñid (P); riṅ (N)
(138) ñuṅs (D & J)
(139) bgrog (N & P)
(140) spyad gis (P)
(141) nu (P)
(142) tsi daṅ not available in (D & J)
(143) gar (N & P)
(144) bźag (N & P)
(145) rtsol (N & P)
(146) khor (N)

APPENDIX - I

(Ka)

		1
ka tsam	वन्यमुद्ग	wild-oat; 193.
ku śu	सेव	apple; 34.
kun	सर्व, निखल	all, the whole; 10,26,32,37,172.
Ke'u	गृंजनक	carrot;173, 176.
klu-sgrub	नागार्जुन	n. of a saint, who propounded Mādhyamika school of Buddhist philosophy, n. of other Buddhist saints also; 1 (F.N.), 206.
Klu-sgrub-sñiṅ-po	नागार्जुन–हृदय नागार्जुन-गर्भ	n. of Buddhist saints; 206.
klog pa	पठन	study ; 127.
dkar po	शुक्ल	white, pure; 15.
bk'a	शासन	instruction; 116.
bká khrims	राज–नियम	royal commandment; 116.
bkru	स्नान, शोधन, विरेचन प्रक्षालन	bath, cleaning, washing; 60,67,72, 85,91,100, 102,122, 148,149,151.
bkru sman	विरेचन कर्म	purgation ; therapy, purgative; 55,83,102,148.
bkres (pa)	क्षुधा	hunger; 135.
rkaṅ pa	पाद	foot; 143.
skad	भाषा	language; 2.
skabs skabs	कदाकदा, वारम्वार	at times frequently; 99.

---

1 Numbers given here are the line-numbers of the text in which Tibetan terms appear. Arranged in Tibetan alphabetical order.

skam (pa)	शुष्क	dry, arid; 28, 180.
skam sa	जांगल भूमि	arid region, dry land; 28.
skigs pa	हिक्का	hiccup; 136.
skems pa	कृश	thin, lean; 13.
skom	पिपासा	thirst; 135,158,162.
skya reṅ	प्रत्यूष	dawn, early morning; 150
sky reṅs śar (ba)	प्रत्यूष प्रथम भाग	first part of down, early morning; 150.
skyid (pa)	सुख	happiness; 205.
skyu ru ra	आमलकी	n. of a medicinal plant : *Emblica officinalis,* Emblic myrobalan; 33, 100.
skyug (pa)	वमन	emesis; 55, 103, 148
skyug sman	वमन कर्म	emetic therapy; 55,103,148.
skyur (ba) (po)	अम्ल	sour; 32, 43, 45, 51, 58, 59, 66, 74, 97, 183.
skye (ba)	उत्पादक, जनक	producer, aggravator; 30,82.
skyed (pa)	जनन	aggravation production; 34, 35, 39, 26, 29 , 31, 32 40-75, 118, 157.
skyer pa	दारुहरिद्रा	n.of a med. plant: *Berberis aristata;* 145.
skyer pái kha ṇḍa	दार्वीरसांजन	ext. from *Berberis; aristata;* 145.
skyes (pa)	जात, जनन	birth, production; 46,199.
skyes bu	पुरुष	man; 6.
skyo ma	यवागू	gruel; 163.
skyon	दोष	fault, defect; 117, 151.
skyor (ba)	पुनः	again, repetition; 109.
skran	गुल्म	phantom tumour; 168, 176, 189.
bska (ba)	कषाय	astringent; 37,42,44,56.
bsku	अभ्यंग, लेप	massage, rubbing; 72,99,143, 145, 149.
bskol (ba)	कषाय, क्वाथ, शृत	boiled, decoction; 65, 72, 100.
bskyed	कारक, उत्पादक	producer; 54,204.
bskyod (pa)	व्यायाम	physical exercise; 60.

(Kha)

kha	मुख	mouth, face; 137,151.
kha ṇḍa	खण्ड	solid ext. in the form of paste; 145
kha (ba)	तिक्त	bitter; 35,43,44,51,84,87,181.
kha ra (ka ra)	शर्करा	sugar; 58,65,86.
khaṅ (ba)	गृह	house; 101.
khu chu	शुक्र	semen; 134.
khu ba	(1) रस	(1) soup; 96, 159.
	(2) शुक्र	(2) semen; 134.
khu tshan	उष्ण रस	hot soup; 159.
khuṅ	कुण्ड	pit, place of workship; 125.
khum	अश्लील	vulgar; 111.
khyim	गृहपालित	domesticated; 189-191.
khyim bya	गृहकुक्कुट	domesticated fowl ;189-191.
khyud (pa)	पूजन	worship; 201.
khyed pa	विशेषतया	specially, particularly; 11,25.
khrag,	रक्त	blood; 83.
khrag dbyuṅ pa	रक्तमोक्षण	bloodletting therapy; 83.
khro (ba)	क्रोध	anger; 9,14.
mkhris pa	पित्त	bile, one of the three morbid factors; 7, 9, 14, 18, 21-24, 26, 30-35, 37, 39-41, 46, 48,51, 82, 106.
'khor	परिवार	family members, attendants; 156, 201.
'khru ba	अतिसार	diarrhoea; 191.

(Ga)

ga gon	कर्कोटी	cucumber; 174.
gaṅ	किंचित्	whatsoever; 110, 164, 184.
yaṅ	यत्किंचित्	whatsoever; 164, 184.
gad mo	हास्य	laughter; 132.
gar mthun	उपयुक्त	suitable, appropriate; 105.
goṅ du	अग्रे	ahead of; 118.

goms (pa)	अभ्यास	habit; 195; 204.
gos	वस्त्र	cloth; 91, 95, 155.
gyur pa	आचरण	behaviour, conduct, to become; 79.
grags pa	यश, कीर्ति	fame; 202.
graṅ (ba)	शीत	cold; 18, 61, 65, 71, 94, 103.
grib ma	छाया	shade; 61, 124.
gro	गोधूम	wheat; 27, 56.
grog	(1) नदीतट	(1) river bank ravine; 129.
	(2) शीतल	(2) cold; 185.
grogs	मित्र	friend; 90, 112.
glal (ba)	जृम्भा	yawning; 137.
dgag (pa)	अवरोध	suppression, inhibition; 135.
dgab (pa)	आवरण	cover; 137.
dgar (dga' bar)	सुख	pleasure, contentment; 199.
dgun	शीतकाल	winter season; 23, 24, 94, 103, 104, 177.
dgun stod	हेमन्त	early winter; 23, 24, 94, 103, 177.
dgun smad	शिशिर	late winter; 23, 94, 103.
dge (ba)	कल्याण	auspiciousness; 112, 204, 205.
dge bcu	दश मंगलकारक कर्म	ten auspicious duties; 112.
dge (ba) sbyoṅ	श्रमण	religious ascetic; 119.
dge bśes (pa)	कल्याण मित्र	auspicious friend; 112.
dge sloṅ	भिक्षु	monk; 118.
dgoṅs pa	भावना, अभिप्राय	thought, purpose; 12.
dgod (pa)	परिहास	jest, joke; 132.
dgon pa	अरण्य	forest, wild; 123.
bgo (ba)	परिधान	to put on or wear cloth; 91, 95.
bgrad (pa)	अनावरण	to keep uncovered, to keep open; 137.
mgo (bo)	शिरस्	head; 99, 139, 143, 146, 148.
mgyogs (pa)	शीघ्र	quickly; 186.
'gam (pa)	भक्षण	eating; 160.
'gom (pa)	अतिक्रमण	to cross, to walk-over; 124.
'gyur (ba)	जनन, प्राप्ति, उत्पन्न	to produce, to cause, to obtain; 167, 174-176, 188, 189.

'graṅs pa	उदरपूर्ण	bellyful; 96, 161, 162, 165.
'gran (pa)	प्रतिस्पर्धा	competition; 117.
'grus (pa)	उत्साह	enthusiasm; 157.
'greṅ (ba)	उत्थान	to stand; 133.
'gro (ba)	गमन	to go, to walk; 78, 89, 118, 131.
rgan po	वृद्ध	old, senior; 17, 131, 163.
rgas (pa)	जरा	old age, aging process; 153.
rgun chaṅ	द्राक्षासव	alcoholic drink prepared of grapes; 57.
rgun ('brum)	द्राक्षा	grapes; 57.
rgod	विचलित	to become wild, agitated; 13.
rgya	(1) देश	(1) country, vast expanse; 2.
	(2) हरिण	(2) dee; 177.
Rgya gar	भारत	India; 2.
Rgya gar skad	संस्कृत भाषा	Sanskrit language; 2.
rgya sran nag po	कृष्णधान्य, माष	black gram; 185.
rgyan	अलंकार	ornament; 92, 155.
rgyam tsha	सामुद्र लवण	sea-salt; 41.
rgyal po	राजा	king, ruler; 114, 115.
rgyal mtshan	ध्वज	flag; 124.
rgyo	रमण, मैथुन	to indulge in sex; 131.
sga	आर्द्रक, शुण्ठी	ginger; 57.
sga chu	शुण्ठ्युदक	ginger water; 57.
sgo ṅa	अण्ड	egg; 190.
sgog skya	लशुन	garlic; 190.
sgor	परिधि	compound; 129.
sgyu ma	माया, विकार	perversion, illusion; 116.
sgra	संगीत	music, song; 67.
bsgrub (sgrub pa)	साधन	practice; 203.
bsgrus	प्रेरण	to incite; 135.

(Na)

ṅa rgyal	अहंकार	ego, pride, arrogance; 111.
ṅag	कथा, वाणी	speech, advice; 130.
ṅad	वायु	air; 18, 69.

ṅad can	वातल	airy, windy; 18.
ṅal ba	आयास, श्रम, व्यायाम	fatigue, exercise; 63, 79, 98.
ṅud mo	क्रन्दन	crying; 132.
ṅes (pa)	निश्चय	to ensure; 73.
ṅoms pa	सन्तोष	satisfaction; 158.
mṅar (ba)	मधुर	sweet; 26, 34, 42, 45, 50, 51, 59, 74, 83, 84, 87, 97.
lṅa bcu lṅa	पंचपचाशत्	fifty five; 201, 203.
sṅags	मंत्र	sacred incantation; 146.
sṅar	पूर्व	before; 109,159.
sṅar bya	पूर्वकृत	deeds of the past; 109.

(Ca)

can	युक्त	suffix meaning possessed with; 14, 19.
ci	किमपि, यथा	what, whatever, appropriate; 60 133, 150, 204.
ci ran,	यथायोग्य	whatever appropriate, appropriately; 60.
cig (gcig)	एक	one; 175, 176, 187, 188, 191.
cir	सदा	always; 108.
cuṅ zad	अल्प	a little; 77, 169, 191.
gci (ba)	मूत्र	urine; 134.
gcig	एक	one; 47, 164, 181.
gcig pa	प्रथम	first; 3.
gcu (ba)	संकोचन	squeezing,contraction; 136.
bcag	(1) चंक्रमण	(1) walking; 60.
	(2) भंग	(2) breaking; 125.
	(3) प्रदर्शन	(3) exhibition; 133.
bcad (pa)	(1) कर्त्तन	(1) cutting; 123.
	(2) रचन	(2) composition; 207.
bca' (ba)	(1) निवास	(1) to reside; 129.
	(2) भक्षण	(2) to chew (for brushing); 151.

bcas	सह	alongwith; 10.
bcu	दश	ten; 112, 199, 200.
lci (ba)	गुरु	heavy; deep, 15, 42, 50, 52, 58, 88, 159.
lce myaṅ tsha	स्फुटिका	alum; 41.

(Cha)

cha	भाग	part; 170.
cha mñam	समभाग	equal part; 170.
chags (pa)	स्नेह, अनुराग	love, attachment; 113, 195.
chaṅ	मद्य	alcoholic drink; 39, 57, 64, 77, 88, 98, 161, 171, 180, 183.
chaṅ Chu	सुरामण्ड	upper layer of the alcoholic drink; 171.
chaṅ rñiṅ	पुराण मद्य	old wine, old alcoholic drink, 57.
chad (pa)	(1) पश्चात्ताप	(1) repentance; 109.
	(2) संध्या	(2) evening; 126.
	(3) सन्यास	(3) to be free from worldly bondage; 203.
cham pa	प्रतिश्याय	cold, influenza; 149.
char pa	वर्षा	rain; 68, 78.
chu	(1) जल	(1) water; 34, 55, 57, 60, 67, 72, 77, 85, 91, 100, 122, 148, 173, 180, 185.
	(2) मण्ड	(2) upper layer; 171.
chu grog	(1) नदीजल	river water; 77.
	(2) शीतल जल	cold water; 185.
chu (dro)'jam	उष्णोदक, सुखोदक	tepid water, slightly warm water; 91.
chu bya	जलकुक्कुट	water fowl; 173.
chu mig	झर	spring, fountain; 122.
chu tsha(n)	उष्णजल	hot water; 55, 60, 148.
chuṅ	अल्प	a little, small; 15, 171.
che (ba)	महत्, अतिमात्र	much, in excess; 14, 97, 111, 132, 164, 171.

ched	निमित्त	because of; 203.
chen po	अधिक, महान्, बृहत्	more, in excess big; 110, 120.
chos	धर्म	religion; 108, 116, 117, 203.
mchi ma	अश्रु	tears; 134.
mchin pa	यकृत्	liver; 169.
mchu	ओष्ठ	lip; 139.
mchog	श्रेष्ठ, अग्र, परम, उत्तम	the best, excellent; 5, 152, 170, 173.
mchod rten	चैत्य	religious monument; 120, 124.
mchod (pa)	प्रार्थना, पूजन	prayer; 120, 124, 155.
'chi ba	मृत्यु	death; 175.
'cho	आयुस	life; 107.

(Ja)

ji ltar	यथा	in whatsoever manner; 48.
'jam	मृदु	soft; 45, 58.
'ju (ba)	पाक	digestion; 196.
'ju sla (ba)	सुपाच्य	easily digestible; 196.
rje dpon	गुरु	preceptor; 157.
rjes	अनन्तर	after wards, 162, 165, 171, 185.
brjod (pa)	निगदित, कथित	stated, described, 12, 25, 117, 156.

(Ña)

ña	मत्स्य	fish; 181, 182, 189.
ñam	भय	fear; 110.
ñal po	व्यवाय, मैथुन, निद्रा, शयन	sexual intercourse, sleep; 62, 80, 127, 136, 165.
ñal (ba)	निद्रा	sleep; 121, 129, 197.
ñi che	प्रदेश	place of habitation; 12.
ñi ma	(1) दिवस (2) सूर्य	(1) day; 21, 95, 126. (2) sun; 128.
ñi ma phyed	मध्याह्न	midday; 21, 126.
ñi śu	विशंति	twenty; 200.
ñid	आत्मन्	self; 46.

ñin par log	दिवानिद्रा	sleep during day time; 59.
ñin (mo) (pa)	दिवा	da; 59, 68, 80, 92.
ñuṅ (ba)	अल्प	a little; 64, 196.
ñe śiṅ	(?)	n. of a med. plant; 29.
ñer bsam	यथायोग्य भावना	appropriate respect; 114.
ñes pa	दोष	morbid factors in the body; 38.
ñon moṅs (pa)	क्लेश	misery, trouble; 5.
gñan pa	चण्ड, क्रूर	fearful, powerful; 122.
gñid	निद्रा	sleep; 15, 68, 135.
gñid kyis log	निद्रा	sleep; 68.
gñis	द्वय	two; 16, 62, 70, 82, 104, 189, 191.
mñan (pa)	श्रवण	to hear; 114, 119, 130.
mñam	सम	equal; 170, 171.
mñe (mñed pa)	अभ्यंग	massage; 60, 72, 99.
rñiṅ (d) (pa)	पुराण	old, over matured; 28, 57, 170, 180, 184.
sñan	श्रवण	to hear; 67, 156.
sñan mñan	सभक्ति श्रवण	to hear with devotion; 67.
sñiṅ gzer	(?)	n. of a med. plant; 27.
sñoms	साम्योत्पादक	to maintain harmony or equilibrium; 29, 38.
brñs pa	अवज्ञा	to show disrespect; 115.

(Ta)

til	तिल	sessame; 73, 89, 99, 142, 144.
tog,	कर्तन	harvest; 97.
gdaṅ (ba)	सेवन, प्रयोग	to resort to; administration, 83, 102, 148.
gtam	प्रवचन	religious speech ; 202.
gtar ka (ga)	शिराव्यध	venesection 83; 103.
gti mug	मोह	illusion, ignorance; 9.
gtum (po)	क्रोध	anger; 117.
gtoṅ (ba)	शुभदान	auspicious charity; 112.
gtoṅ (pa)	प्रणिपात	submission; 119.

gtor ma	बलि	sacrificial offering; 125.
btaṅ	प्रयोग	administration; 55.
btab	मिश्रण, युक्त,	addd, mixed, afflicted; 65, 149.
btuṅ (ba)	आक्रान्त पान	to drink; 55, 57, 64, 77, 87, 88, 98, 127, 161, 162.
rta	अश्व	horse; 165, 187.
rta rgyug (pa)	अश्वारोहण	horse-riding; 165.
rtag (tu)	सदा	always; 84, 133, 143, 146, 152, 195.
rtags	प्रकृति, लक्षण	characteristic features, signs; 12.
rtog (pa)	तर्क	argument; 117.
rtogs (pa)	ज्ञान	knowledge, known; 120.
lta (ba)	दर्शन	to look; 17.
lto (ba)	उदर	abdomen; 188.
lto'i srin bu	उदरकृमि	worms in abdomen; 188.
sta rka	अक्षोट	walnut; 27.
staṅ zil;	रसांजन	antimony; 145.
stan	आसन	seat; 101.
stan gdiṅ	आस्तरण	carpet; 81.
stug	स्थुल	thick; 101.
stegs	वेदी	seat for the gods and saints; 125.
stoṅ (pa)	शून्यस्थान	empty house; 120.
stod	पूर्व	first part; 22, 23, 62, 176.
ston	शरत्	autumn; 22, 24, 82, 142, 144.
stobs	साहस	exhibition of strength; 79, 165.
brta (ba)	विस्तार	to expand; 163.
brag (pa)	परीक्षा	examination; 19.
brtun (pa)	अतिक्लान्त	excessive exhaustion; 80.
brtul zugs (can)	मुनि	ascetic sage; 6.
blta	दर्शन	to look; 128.
bstan	प्रदर्शन	to exhibit; 156.
bstan pa	शासन, आख्यान, उपदेश	explanation, instruction; 8, 25, 49, 107.
bsten	उपभोग, सेवन, प्रदर्शन	to enjoy, to attend, to exhibit; 90, 112, 130.

(Tha)

thag	गत	to become, to pass over; 172.
Thams cad mkhyen pa	सर्वज्ञ	Omniscient; 4.
thal khun	भस्मकुण्ड	place of sacred ashes; 125.
thal ba	भस्म	ashes; 125.
thug pa	यूष	vegetable soup; 159.
tho rans	प्रत्यूष	dawn; 20.
thob pa	प्राप्त	to obtain; 8, 205.
thos (pa)	श्रवण	to hear; 204.
mthil	तल	bottom, sole (of foot); 143.
mthun pa	अनुकुल	beneficial; 48, 114.
'thun (s)	पान	to drink; 65, 85, 158, 163, 171, 174, 179, 185.

(Da)

dar	यौवन	youth; 17.
dar cus bslad	जलमिश्रित तक्र	butter-milk mixed with water; 37.
dar (ra) (pa)	तक्र	butter-milk; 34, 65.
dug	विष	poison; 85, 170.
dug med	निर्विष	free from poison; 85.
dugs	स्वेदन	fomentation therapy; 73, 104.
dud pa	धूम	smoke; 147.
dub pa	(1) मन्द (2) क्लान्त	(1) mild; 79. (2) fatigue; 131.
dur khrod	श्मशान	cemetery, crematorium; 121.
dur (ba)	शव	dead body; 121.
dus	काल, समय	time; season, 10, 20, 21, 25, 47, 53, 54, 62, 82, 85, 102, 142, 144, 158.
de	तत्	that; 49, 100, 105, 150, 152, 156, 195, 198.
de rjes	तदनन्तर	thereafter; 100.

de ltaṅ	तथा	like that; 195.
de ltar	तथा	like that; 105, 198, 205.
de nas	तदनन्तर	thereafter; 152, 156, 200, 201.
de phyir	तदर्थ	for that; 49.
de riṅ	तत्काल	at that time; 150.
de las	तदनन्तर	thereafter; 16.
des (pa)	पेशल, भद्र	gentle, noble conduct; 113, 198.
don	अर्थ	meaning, object; 8, 140, 147, 205.
dor ba	त्याग	to throw out; 109.
drag tu	सशक्त, तीव्र	violently, strong; 139, 167.
drag po	रुद्र, अति, गरिमा, क्रूर	fierceful, sharp, inexcess; 69, 88, 130, 132, 147.
drag po'i ṅad	वात्या	strong wind; 69.
drag śul	अतिव्यायाम	vigorous exercise; 62, 79.
drags	अतिमात्र	excessively; 177, 178.
draṅ (ba)	आकर्षण, उत्क्लेश	attraction, to draw out; 55.
draṅ sroṅ,	ऋषि	sage; 6, 119.
draṅ sroṅ chen po	महर्षि	great sage; 11.
daṅs	शीर्ण	emaciation; 168.
dri	गन्ध	smell; 14, 147.
dri ma	मल	dirt; 91.
dri ma med	निर्मल	clean; 91.
dri źim (pa)	सुगन्ध	agreeable smell; 92.
drug	षट्	six; 25, 164.
druṅ	निकट	near; 120.
dro	भोजन	meal; 159.
dro (ba)	उष्ण	hot; 27, 30, 32, 36, 40, 50, 51, 61, 67, 69, 93, 195.
dro bab	भोजन ग्रहण	to take meal; 159.
dro min	अनुष्ण	not hot; 69, 93.
drod	ऊष्मा, दीपन	heat, digestive stimulant; 14, 15, 75, 97, 159.
dron po	उष्ण	hot; 76, 101, 172.
gdags	परिधान, वहन, धारण	to wear, to carry; 67, 92, 141, 146.
gduṅ (ba)	तप्त	to be scorched; 18.
gdoṅ	मुख	face; 151.

bdag	आत्मन्	self; 157.
bdud rtsi	अमृत	ambrosia; 152.
bde (ba)	सुख	happiness; 10, 80, 92, 197, 204.
mdo	सूत्र	rule, axiom, statement in brief; 1, 2, 207.
mdoṅs (pa)	आन्ध्य	blindness; 177.
mdor	संदेश, संक्षेप	in brief; 25.
'di	अयं, अत्र	this, here; 12, 49, 85, 154, 184.
'di rnams	एते	these; 184.
'dug (pa)	निवास, विश्राम, उपवेशन	to stay, to remain, to sit; 61, 69, 78, 81, 89, 101, 133, 150.
'dod (pa)	काम, इच्छा	lust, sensual desire; 9, 110, 117.
'dom	वर्णन	description; 47.
'dra,	स्वयं	self; 46.
'de (ba)	मिश्रण	mixture; 174.
'dres pa	मिश्रित	mixed; 19.
rdul	धुलि	dust 110.
rdo	पाषाण	stone; 123.
ldaṅ (ba)	उत्थान, कारक, संक्रमण, प्रकोप	to arise, to produce, to get aggravated; 22, 23, 47, 48, 54, 70, 81, 82, 164, 166, 168.
ldam ldum	निन्ध	not useful; 166, 167.
ldum	शाक	vegetable; 173.
ldum mchag	उत्तमशाक	best among vegetables; 173
sdig (pa)	पाप, अशुभ	sinful, inauspicious; 112.
sdod	काम	passion; 95.
brdab (pa)	पीडन	to press, to squeeze; 139, 140.
brdos (pa)	भर्जित	fried; 192.

(Na)

na	यदा	when, if; 71.
na le śam	मरिच	black pepper: *Piper nigrum*; 31, 66.
nag po	कृष्ण	black; 185.
naṅ	अन्तः	inside; 94, 163, 192.
naṅ nub	पश्चात्	afterwards; 109.

nan par	प्रातः	morning; 20.
nad	व्याधि, रोग	disease, malady, sickness; 5, 47, 54, 71-73, 82, 104, 105, 135, 164, 166-168, 172.
nad can	रोगी	patient; 168.
nan tan	उद्यम	professional duty; 157, 198.
nam	रात्रि	night; 21, 197.
nam sros	रात्रि	night; 197.
nam mkha'	आकाश	sky; 126.
nas	(1) अनन्तर	(1) thereafter; 25.
	(2) यव	(2) barley; 28, 56, 86.
nub	पश्चात्	afterwards; 109.
nub mo	सायं	evening; 180.
nus (pa)	शक्ति	strength, ability; 133, 140, 205.
gnag (pa)	(1) अवरोध	(1) obstruction, inhibition; 135.
	(2) चर्मरी	(2) yak, black cattle; 176, 187, 188.
gnas	स्थान, आवास, गृह	place of habitation, house; 12, 53, 61, 69, 81, 93, 101, 129, 156, 204.
gnod (pa)	दुषित, पीडा, अहितकर	vitiation, harm, injury; 38, 41, 113, 166, 169, 170, 171, 174, 182, 184, 185, 192, 196.
gnon (pa)	पान	to drink; 180.
mnan	रोध	to subdue; 141.
rna (ba)	कर्ण	ear; 144.
rno (ba)	तीक्ष्ण	sharp, pointed; 14.
sna	(1) शिखर	(1) top, peak; 129.
	(2) नासा	(2) nose; 144.
sna tshogs	विविध	different types; 98.
snabs	सिंघाणक	nasal secretion; 134.
snar	विस्तार	expansion; 129.
snum pa	स्निग्ध, स्नेह	unctuous, oil, etc.;15, 50, 52, 58, 72, 96, 149, 159.
snum bag	स्निग्धभोजन	unctuous food; 19, 96.
snod	भाण्ड	vessel; 181.

(Pa)

dpyad (dpyod pa)	परीक्षा	examination, investigation; 12.
dpyas (pa)	द्वेष	to find fault with others; 117.
dpyid	वसन्त	spring; 22, 54, 142, 144.
spaṅ(s) (ba)	त्याग	to give up, to avoid; 62, 66, 77, 80, 103, 110, 112, 127, 132, 165, 169, 173, 180.
spyad	आचरण, सेवन, उपभोग	enjoyment; 7, 53, 112.
spyi brtol	घृणा, निर्लज्ज	hatred, shamelessness; 111.
spyod chul	चर्या	conduct, 47.
spyod lam	चर्या, आचरण	conduct, manner, behaviour; 7, 52, 107, 116.
spri	पीतभाग	yalk, yellow part of the egg; 190.
spugs	कम्पन	to shake; 139.

(Pha)

pha	पिता	father; 118.
pha boṅ	बृहत् पाषाण	big boulder; 123.
phag pa	वराह	boar; 188.
phag tshun	परस्पर	with each other; 138.
phan pa	हित	beneficial; 48, 65, 68, 85, 154.
phug (pa)	गुफा	cave; 120.
pho ba,	आमाशय	stomach; 75.
phog ('phog pa)	सम्पृक्त	to come in contact; 147, 166.
phyag 'tshal (ba)	नमस्	to bow before; 4, 5, 6.
phyi	वहिस्	outside; 94.
phyi dro	अपराह्ण	afternoon; 20, 197.
phyi rol	बाह्य	outside; 71.
phyin	अग्रे	afterwards; 109, 203.
phyi chad	उपरान्त	thereafter; 203.
phyir	हेतु	reason, because of; 11, 49, 53, 72, 107, 203.

phyis	अनन्तर	afterwards, at the end; 160.
phyugs	प्राणी	animal; 142.
phyugs mar	प्राणिवसा	animal fat; 142.
phye	शक्तु	roasted corn flour; 160, 162.
phyed	अर्ध, मध्य	middle, half; 21.
phra snags	तीक्ष्ण	sharp; 128.
phrom	?	? ; 58.
'phags pa	आर्य	noble; 206.
'phyen	अधोवायु	flatus; 134.
'phrad pa	मिश्रण	mixture; 160.
'phrod pa	सात्म्य, हितकर	wholesome, useful; 7, 36, 48-53,. 106, 175, 178, 181, 184, 193· 195, 197.

(Ba)

bag,	(1) अन्न	(1) food, meal; 59, 63, 75, 79.
	(2) भोजन	(2) intake of food; 7, 95, 97, 198.
bag byed	(1) अधिक भोजन	(1) intake of more food; 97.
	(2) अल्पाधिक	(2) more or less, appropriately; 109, 115.
bag che	संक्षेप	brief; 107.
bag ma	स्त्री	wife; 93.
bań	धावन	running; 165.
bad kan	कफ	one of the three morbid factors in the body; 7, 9, 15, 19, 20, 22· 24, 26, 29, 30, 32, 35, 37, 39, 40, 46, 48, 52, 54, 55, 94, 106.
ban bun	खण्डित	broken; 126.
bab	ग्रहण	to take; 159.
bab chol	शीघ्र	quickly; 161.
bam po	भाग	section, subdivision; 3.
bar	मध्य, अन्तर	between, intermediate period; 199.
bar bar	कदा कदा	at times; 143, 145.

bar 'ga'	अन्तरान्तरा	in between; 75.
bal po se'u	दाडिम	pomegranate; 33.
bu rum	गुड	jaggery; 27, 28, 57, 64, 194.
bu nam rñid	पुराण गुड	old jaggery; 28.
bud med	स्त्री	woman; 130, 131.
bud med rgan	वृद्धा	old woman; 131.
Bod skad	भोट भाषा	Tibetan language; 2.
bya	(1) करण, कर्तव्य	(1) to make, to do; 7, 8, 16, 17, 21, 59, 60, 63, 68, 73, 77, 78, 84, 88, 95, 98, 104, 105, 109, 111, 113, 115, 117, 121, 123, 125, 131, 138, 141, 146, 147, 150, 181, 197, 198, 200.
	(2) पक्षी, कुक्कुट	(2) bird, fowl; 173, 189-191.
bya gag	वक	crane; 194.
byams pa	मैत्री	friendship; 113.
byas (pa)	कृत, परिधान	to do, to wear; 155, 171, 202.
byi dor	मार्जन, शोधन	cleaning; 146.
byis pa	शिशु	child; 17.
byug pa	धारण	to wear; 155.
byed pa	कारक	to do, to perform; 26, 30, 33, 35, 38-41, 110, 204.
bra po	फाफर	buck-wheat; 179.
bri ('bri ba)	दारण	to scratch, to draw; 140.
brud	घर्षण	rubbing; 138.
bregs (pa)	कर्तन	to cut; 138.
bro (ba)	रस	taste; 164.
blugs	मिश्रण, पुरण	mixed, to pour; 76, 144.
blo	मति	mind, intellect, wisdom; 6, 14.
blo ldan pa	मतिमान्	wise person; 6.
dbaṅ bsgyur (ba)	नियमन	to control; 10.
dbab (pa)	प्रवेश	to enter into; 199.
dbugs mibde	श्वास	asthma, dyspnoea; 190.
dbyar	(1) ग्रीष्म	(1) summer; 22, 23, 62, 70, 102, 104, 173.
	(2) ज्येष्ठ	(2) n. of a month (April-May); 167.

dbyar stod	ग्रीष्मपूर्वभाग	first part of summer; 22, 62, 102, 104, 142.
dbyar smad	प्रावृट्, ग्रीष्म पश्चात भाग	later part of summer, 23, 24, 70, 102.
dbyar zla	ज्येष्ठमास	n. of a month (April-May); 167.
dbyuṅ pa	निर्हरण, मोक्षण	to take out; 83.
'byuṅ (ba)	उद्भव, उत्पन्न	to give rise to; 178, 186.
'bras	शालि	rice; 63, 76, 86, 160, 162.
'bras chan	भृष्ट शालि	fried paddy; 76.
'briṅ po	मध्यम	middle, mediocre; 167, 173.
'bru	धान्य	corn, cereal; 97.
sbyaṅ ba	शोधन	cleaning; 99.
sbyar (ba)	मिश्रित	mixed; 36, 48, 74, 164.
sbraṅ chu	मधूदक	water mixed with honey; 57.
sbraṅ caṅ	मध्वासव	alcoholic drink prepared of honey; 57.
sbraṅ rtsi	मधु	honey; 28, 56, 57, 75, 86, 170, 175, 193.
sbrid pa	क्षवथु	sneezing; 134, 137.
sbrul	सर्प	snake; 119.
sbrub pa	साधन	to perform, to do; 114.

(Ma)

ma	(1) माता	(1) mother; 118.
	(2) न	(2) negative; 120, 134, 160, 172, 193.
ma laṅs	तरुण, अपक्व	immature; 172.
ma ṇḍa la	मण्डल	mystic and sacred circle; 124.
ma togs (pa)	व्यतिरिक्त	with the exception of; 6.
ma rtogs	अज्ञात	unknown; 120.
ma thag	सद्य	immediately after maturity; 172.
ma nu	पुष्कर	n. of a med. plant: *Inula racemosa*; 193.
ma nu'i sa bon	पुष्कर बीज	seeds of *Inula racemosa;* 193.
ma źu (ba)	अजीर्ण	indigestion; 149.

maṅ (po) (ba)	बहु, अधिक	more; 13, 39, 121, 166, 179, 182, 184.
mar	(1) स्निग्ध, स्नेह, वसा	(1) unctuous, oil, fat; 45, 58, 75, 96, 142, 153, 170, 178, 181.
	(2) तैल	(2) oil; 73, 89, 99, 192.
mar khu	घृत	ghee, melted butter; 76.
mar rñiṅ	पुराण घृत	old ghee; 170.
mar (g)sar	नवनीत	butter (fresh); 63, 87, 153.
mar 'bri (b) pa	आदान, अपकर्ष	degeneration, decreasing; 62.
mar 'bri dus	आदान काल	time of absorption; 62.
mas	अनुलोमन	downward movement; 42, 44.
mas btaṅ	अनुवासन	a type of medicated enema containing oil, etc.; 73.
mi	(1) मानव	(1) man; 8, 13-15, 92, 113, 125, 198, 199, 205.
	(2) न	(2) negative indicator, not; 29, 34, 38, 41, 48-52, 59, 61, 63, 78, 80, 81, 88, 89, 102, 104, 111, 115-117, 119, 121-125, 127-131, 133, 134, 136-141, 147-149, 161, 162, 171, 175, 178, 181, 194.
mi ldaṅ	रहित	free from; 81.
mi 'phrod (pa)	असात्म्य, अहितकर	unwholesome; 49-52.
mi ro	शव	dead body; 125, 147.
mig	चक्षु	eye; 145, 177.
min	विना, न, अप्राप्त	except, without, no, not being available; 74, 93, 111, 113, 127, 135, 153, 161, 184.
mu ka	मुद्ग	*Phaseolus mungo*; 28.
me	अग्नि	fire; 101.
med	रहित, विपरीत	without, opposite; 69, 74, 81, 85, 91, 107, 110, 140, 160, 196.
med smra (ba)	विपरीत भाषण	negative speaking; 108.
mos (pa)	ओष, तुषार	dew drops; 166.
mya ṅan	दुःख	sorrow; 141.

myur (ba)	शीघ्र	hurridly, quickly; 135.
myos pa	तीव्र, मत्तन्त्_त	strong, intoxicating; 161.
dman	नीच, हीन	mean; 111.
dmar thag	प्रत्यूष	dawn; 126.
dmar (po)	रक्त	red colour; 14.
rma	सौन्दर्य	beauty; 115.
sma	नम्र	humble; 199.
smad	पश्चात्_भाग	later part; 22, 23, 70.
sman	औषध, भैषज्य	medicine, drug; 1, 2, 55, 72, 83, 84 100, 146, 148, 152, 154, 174, 207.
sman mchog	औषधि श्रेष्ठ	the best among medicines; 152.
sman pa	भिषक्	physician; 5, 206.
Sman pa'i mchog	भिषक् श्रेष्ठ	the Best among Physicians: Lord Buddha; 5.
Sman 'tsho ba'i mdo	वैद्य–जीव–सूत्र	n. of this work; 1, 2, 207.
smos	कथन	speech; 112.
smra ba	भाषण	speaking, noise; 108, 131, 137.

(Tsa)

sam	किंचित्_ मात्र	as much as; 8.
si	जुर्णाह्व	millet; 193.
sog bu (pu)	प्रांजलि आसन	squatting with folded hands; 68, 150.
gtsan (ba)	निर्मल, पवित्र	free from impurity; 85.
tson	पालण्डु	onion; 175.
tsal	साहस	exhibition of excessive strength; 131.
tsub (pa)	रुक्ष, परुष	rough, coarse, unctuous; 13, 44, 50, 52, 56.
e (ba)	क्रीडा	play; 119.
sol bcag	सामान्य कर्म	normal work; 99.
rtsam pa	दृष्ट	found; 105.

brtsal ba	कर्तव्य कर्म	professional duty; 200.
brtson pa	प्रयत्न, कर्म	to strive, to make efforts, 157, 204

(Tsha)

tsha (tshwa)	लवण	saline, salt; 58.
tsha (ba)	(1) कटु	(1) pungent; 30, 43, 45, 51.
	(2) उष्ण	(2) hot, heat; 18, 52, 60, 61, 66, 71, 74, 90, 94, 102 181.
tsha min	अनुष्ण	not hot; 74.
tshad	मान	span, measurement; 198.
tshan mo	उष्ण	hot, warm; 55, 159, 185.
tshig	वाक्, वाणी	talk, speech; 13, 15.
tshigs	छन्द, पद्य	metrics, verse; 207.
tshil	मेदस्, वसा	fat; 58, 64, 75, 89, 96, 178, 181.
tshul	चर्या, शील	conduct; 12, 49, 112.
tshe	समय, आयुस्	time, life; 126, 136, 137, 153, 154, 167, 186, 198.
tshe riṅ	दीर्घायुस्	longevity; 153.
tshon	मेदस्वी	fatty; 96.
mtshan	रात्रि	night; 80, 92.
mtsho	ह्रद	lake; 122.
'tsho ba	जीवन, आयुस्	life, support; 1, 2, 8, 198, 207.

(Dza)

Dzi ba sū tra	जीव सूत्र	principle of healthy living, n. of this work; 2.
mdziṅ	ग्रीवा	neck; 136.
mdzes (pa)	सुन्दर	beautiful; 155.
'dzum	स्मित	smiling; 156.
'dzem	त्याग	to avoid, to shun; 108.
rdzogs	समाप्त	completion; 207.
brdzaṅs pa (rdzoṅs pa)	निगदित	to forward, to despatch; 206.

(Źa)

źi ba	शान्ति	to get alleviated, to be pacified; 24.
źu ba	जीर्ण	digestion; 149.
źun mar	घृत	ghee, melted butter; 27, 153.
źes	इति	thus; 10.
źo	दधि	curd; 172, 174, 194.
gźag (pa)	स्थित	to remain; 199.
gźan	अपर	others; 108, 113, 117, 142, 144, 157.
gźom (pa)	भंग	to break; 123.
bźag (pa)	स्थित	to exist, to keep; 138.
bźi	चत्वार	four; 94, 158.
bźin	अनुक्रम, यथा, अनुसार	gradually, according to, like; 45, 141, 170, 198.
bźin rim	अनुक्रम	gradually; 43.
bźugs	विहरण, आसीन, सन्निधान	to remain, to exist; to be contained; 1.

(Za).

zan	भोजन	food, meal; 76, 162, 186.
zan dron	उष्ण भोजन, शक्तु	hot food, roasted corn flour; 76.
zas	अन्न, भोजन	food, meal; 12, 47, 53, 74, 86, 90, 96, 158, 170, 195, 197.
zil ba	तुषार	dew, frost; 89.
zer ma	बिन्दु (?)	drop(?); 182.
zos (za ba)	भक्षण	eating; 152, 154, 164, 169, 170, 171, 175-179, 182, 184, 186-192, 196, 197.
zla (ba)	(1) मास	(1) month; 54, 70, 82, 94, 167, 173.
	(2) चन्द्र	(2) moon; 90, 186.
zla ba spyan kyis zin	चन्द्रग्रहण (?)	lunal eclipse; 186.
gzir ba	अक्रान्त	to suffer, to be afflicted; 104.

gze ma	गोक्षुर	*Tribulus terrestris;* 27.
bzad po	खरस्रोतस्	having strong current; 122.
bza' ba	भोजन	food; 56, 63, 64, 75, 76, 84, 87, 89, 96, 97, 127, 158-161, 167, 178.

('A)

a'ṅ	अपि	even; 95.
o'(ma)	दुग्ध	milk; 63, 65, 87.
o'ṅ (ba)	आगमन, जात	to come, to become; 168, 187.
o'd zer	किरण	ray; 128.

(Ya)

ya mtshan	(1) सिद्ध	(1) mystic; 119.
	(2) हास्य	(2) to ridicule, to play joke; 130.
yaṅ	अपि, यदि	also, if; 16.
yaṅ (po) (ba)	लघु	light; 43, 50, 56, 64, 79, 87, 160.
yi ge	अक्षर	alphabet; 127.
yi ge klog	पठन	study; 127.
yid	मनस्	mind; 90, 114.
yid du o'ṅ	मनोरम	friendly; 90.
yin yaṅ	यत्र	whereever; 105.
yuṅs	सर्षप	mustard, 184; 192.
yuṅs rñiṅ	पुराण सर्षप	old mustard; 184.
yuṅs mar	सर्षपतैल	mustard oil; 192.
yum	मातृ	mother; 203.
yul	देश, स्थान	place of habitation; 10, 18, 19, 25, 47, 90, 116, 202.
yod (pa)	अस्ति, युक्त	to exist; 88, 205.
yos	भृष्टयव	roasted barley; 76.
g'yan pa	कण्डू	itching; 187.
g'yal	जृम्भा	yawning; 134.
g'ya' (ba)	कण्डू	itching; 179.
g'yuṅ druṅ	स्वास्तिक, मंगल	auspicious; 15.

g'yer (ma)	वन्यमरिच	wild capsicum; 169, 177.
g'yos pa	आक्रान्त	attacked; 71.

(Ra)

ra ro	मत्त	intoxicated; 88.
raṅ	आत्मन्, स्वयं	self; 53, 107, 110, 199.
raṅ ñam	आत्मभय	fear complex; 110.
ran (pa)	सम्यक्, मित, सम, यथायोग्य	appropriate; 39, 60, 61, 74, 98, 133, 158, 163, 164.
ran dro	सुखोष्ण	luke-warm, 61, 67.
ram ñe	नीली	indigo: *Indigofera tinctoria*; 29.
ri	पर्वत	mountain; 129.
ri boṅ	शश	rabbit; 191.
rig pa	ज्ञान	to know; 204.
rigs pa	विद्या	knowledge; 108.
riṅ	(अधिक) काल	long time; 132, 133, 138, 150, 153.
riṅ riṅ	अतिकाल	long time; 128.
rin chen	मणि	gems and jewels; 146.
rim	अनुक्रम	respectively, successively; 17.
rim b'zin	क्रमशः	consecutively, gradually; 42, 44.
rims	ज्वर, संक्रामक रोग	fever, infectious disease; 174.
rus (pa)	अस्थि	bone; 96.
rus khu	अस्थिरस	bone-soup; 96.
reg (pa)	स्पर्श	to touch, to expose; 68.
res 'ga'	कदाकदा	at times; 144.
ro	(1) रस	(1) taste; 25, 88.
	(2) मृत शरीर	(2) dead body; 125.
ro yod	रसयुक्त	delicious; 88.
rlan	आर्द्र	humid, moist; 19, 78, 81, 95.
rluṅ	वायु	one of the three morbid factors; 7, 9, 13, 18, 20, 22-24, 26, 31, 32, 35-37, 39, 40, 46, 48, 50, 70, 72, 73, 81, 106, 109.
rlon (pa)	आर्द्र	wet, green, moist; 183.

(La)

la phug	मूलक	radish; 180, 183, 194.
la phug rñid	जीर्णमूलक	over matured radish; 180.
la sogas pa	प्रमुख, इत्यादि	etcetera, and others, 10, 49, 56, 58, 66, 86, 100, 128, 136, 154, 159, 160, 165, 183.
lag pa	हस्त	hand; 139, 140, 151.
laṅ tshe	यौवन	youth; 196.
laṅs (laṅ ba)	उत्तिष्ठन, उत्थित, पक्व	to get up, matured; 151, 172.
lan tshwa	लवण	salt; 40, 42, 44, 66, 97.
lam	पथ, मार्ग	road; 120, 203.
lam mdo	चतुष्पथ	cross-road; 120.
las	कर्म	work; 98, 127, 157, 197.
lug	मेष	sheep; 153.
lug gi mar	मेषवसा	sheep-fat; 153.
luṅ	आदेश आगम	instructions, command; 114.
lud pa	कास	coughing; 134, 136.
lums	अवगाह	medicated bath; 73, 104, 168.
lus	शरीर	body; 8, 10, 13, 25, 47, 53, 60, 67, 71, 72, 78, 91, 92, 99, 105, 136, 139, 143, 146, 148, 149, 154, 163, 179, 187, 192, 204, 205.
lo	वर्ष	year; 199, 200.
log	(1) विपरीत	(1) opposite; 59.
	(2) निद्रा	(2) sleep; 59, 68, 80.
loṅ spyod	काम, भागे	passion, enjoyment; 111, 202.
loṅ (pa)	प्रवेश	to enter, to arrive at; 200, 201, 203.

(Śa)

śa	मांस	meat, 28, 57, 63, 76, 86, 96, 174, 176, 180, 187-189, 191, 194.
śa skam	शुष्कमांस	dry-meat, 180.

śa pa	मृग	large-stag; 174.
śa mo	छत्रक	mushroom; 192.
śaṅ tshe	(?)	(?); 183.
śar (ba)	पूर्वभाग, प्रथम भाग	early part; 150.
śiṅ	वृक्ष, काष्ठ	tree, twig; 120, 123, 151.
śiṅ chen	महावृक्ष	big tree; 123.
śiṅ tog	फल	fruit; 166, 183.
śin du (tu)	अत्यन्त	excessively, very much; 155.
śin du mrdzes (pa)	अतिसुन्दर	very beautiful; 155.
śu dag	वचा	*Acorus calamus;* 36.
śu ba	विद्रधि, विस्फोटक	abscess, blister; 186.
śed	कथन	statement, speaking; 111.
śes pa	ज्ञान	to know; 16, 17, 21, 129.
gśer ba	सिक्त	to get drenched; 78.
bśaṅ (ba)	पुरीष	stool; 134.
bśal ba	प्रक्षालन	to wash; 122.
bśes pa	मित्र	friend; 112.

(Sa)

sa	भूमि, स्थान	land, region; 18, 28, 121, 140.
sa bon	बीज	seed; 193.
su	भद्र	auspicious; 205.
sum cu rtsa lṅa	पंचत्रिंश	thirty five; 201.
sen mo	नख	nail; 138.
sems	चित्त, मनस्, सत्व, प्राण	mind, spirit, life; 13, 121, 204.
sems can	प्राणी	animal; 121.
sems can maṅ du bsad pa	अधिक प्राणी वध	slaughter of many animals; 121.
ser ka	पीत	yellow; 14.
ser bu	करका, शीतवात	hail-stone, cold wind; 69, 147.
sel (ba)	अपनयन, निराकरण, प्रशमन	to cleanse, to remove, to cure, to alleviate; 5, 26, 29-33, 35-37, 73.

so	(1) दन्त	(1) tooth; 151, 186.
	(2) सुख	(2) happiness; 178.
so na śu ba	दन्तविद्रधि	gum abscess, tumour in tooth; 186.
so śiṅ	दन्तकाष्ठ	twig for brushing teeth; 151.
sra ba	सारत्व	compactness; 153.
sran ma	शिम्बीधान्य	pulses; 86.
sras	कुमार	son; 115.
sri	सम्मान	respect; 118.
sri zu ba	पूज्य मित्र	respected friend; 118, 156.
srid	(1) नियमन	(1) govern; 9.
	(2) अरोग	(2) to climb a hight; 202.
srin bu	कृमि	worm; 188.
srog chags	प्राणी	animal; 31, 119.
srod	सांय	dusk; 20.
sros	सन्ध्या	evening; 197.
sla	सुकर, कर्तव्य	easy work, duty; 98, 104.
sle tres	गुडूची	*Tinospora cordifolia*; 36.
slo	मल	stool; 121.
sloṅ	उत्पन्न	to give rise to, to cause; 172.
slob dpon	आचार्य	preceptor; 118, 206.
gsar tog	नव	freshly harvested; 97.
gsil (ba)	शीत	cold; 59.
gsuṅs	कथन	statement, speech; 11.
gsum (ka)	त्रय	three; 7, 9, 38, 42-46, 71, 106, 108.
gsog (pa)	संचय	accumulation; 22, 23, 70, 94.
gsoṅ (pa)	पूर्वाभिभाषी	to wish in advance; 113.
bsad pa	वध	killing; 121.
bsam (pa)	चिन्तन	to think; 109, 114, 150.
bsal	प्रशम, शोधन, उद्घाटन	alleviation, release, cleanse; 72, 135, 151.
bsil (ba)	शीत	cooling; 26, 34, 35, 37, 50-52, 59, 69, 81, 83, 84, 93, 160.
bser bu	वात	wind; 93.
bser bu mi phog	निवात	free from wind; 93.
bsod pa	उत्तम	the best, agreeable; 163.

bsruṅ (ba)	रक्षण, पालन	protection, to follow; 116.
bsre ba	मिश्रण	mixture; 196.
bsregs (pa)	दग्ध	burnt; 175.
bsro khaṅ	उष्ण गृह	heated house, warm residence; 101.
bsro (ba)	उष्ण	hot; 101.
bsreg (pa)	भर्जित	fried, roasted; 56.
bslad (pa)	मिश्रण	mixed, adulterated; 34.
bslab	शिक्षा	education; 200.
bslu (ba)	अपचिन्तन	deception; 116.

(Ha)

ha caṅ	अधिक	more; 61, 74, 137, 161.
hom khuṅ	हामकुण्ड	place for sacrificial offerings; 125.
lha	देव	god; 114, 155.
lha khaṅ	मन्दिर	temple; 129.
lha (ba)	पूति, पुरण	stale, putrified, preserved for a long time; 178.
lhags	आगमन	advent; 95.
lhan	सह	alongwith; 175, 176, 182, 187-189, 191.
lhan cig	एकत्र	together; 175, 176, 182, 187-189, 191.

(A)

a ru ra	हरतिकी	*Terminalia chebula*; 38, 152.
ā rya	आचार्य	preceptor; 124.

APPENDIX—II

अ

अक्षर	yi ge	alphabet
अक्षोट	sta rka	walnut
अग्नि	me	fire
अग्रे	phyin	(1) that which is to arrive, afterwards
	goṅ du	(2) ahead of
अजीर्ण	ma źu (ba)	indigestion
अज्ञात	ma rtogs	unknown
अण्ड	sgo ṅa	egg
अति	drag po	in excess
अतिकाल	riṅ riṅ	long time
अतिक्रमण	'gom (pa)	to cross, to walk over
अतिक्लान्त	brtun (pa)	excessively tiring efforts
अतिमात्र	(1) drags (2) cheba	excessively
अतिव्यायाम	drag'sul	vigorous exercise
अतिसार	'khru ba	diarrhoea
अतिसुन्दर	śin tu mdzes (pa)	very beautiful
अत्यन्त	śin du (tu)	excessively
अथा च	de ltaṅ (de ltar yaṅ)	like that
अधिक	(1) chen (po) (2) ha caṅ	more, in excess, big
अधिक प्राणि वध	sems can maṅ du bsad pa	slaughter of many animals
अधिक भोजन	bag che	more food
अधोवायु	'phyen	flatus

अनन्तर	(1) nas	case sign indicating thereafter
	(2) rjas	afterwards
	(3) phyis	at the end
अनावरण	bgrad (pa)	to keep uncovered, to keep wide-opened
अनुकूल	mthun pa	beneficial
अनुक्रम	(1) bźin rim	gradually
	(2) rim	successively, respectively
	(3) bźin	accordingly
अनुरक्त	chags (pa)	attachment
अनुलोमन	mas	downward movement
अनुवासन	mas btaṅ	a type of medicated enema
अनुष्ण	(1) tsha min	not hot
	(2) dro min	
अनुसार	bźin	accordingly
अन्तः	naṅ	inside
अन्तर	bar	between
अन्तरान्तरा	bar 'ga'	in between
अन्न	(1) bag	food
	(2) zas	
अन्य	gźan	other
अपकर्ष	mar 'bri(ba) pa	degeneration
अपकार	gnod (pa)	injury, harm
अपक्व	ma laṅs	immature
अपचिन्तन	bslu (ba)	deception
अपनयन	sel (ba)	to cleanse, to cure
अपर	gźan	other
अपराह्न	phi dro	afternoon
अपि	(1) a'ṅ	even, also
	(2) yaṅ	
अप्राप्त	min	not being available
अभिप्राय	dgoṅs pa	purpose
अभ्यंग	(1) bsku	massage, rubbing
	(2) mñe (mñed pa)	
अभ्यास	goms (pa)	habit

अमृत	bdud rtsi	ambrosia
अम्ल	skyur (ba) (po)	sour
अयं	'di	this
अरण्य	dgon pa	forest, wild
अर्थ	don	meaning, object
अर्ध	phyed	half, middle
अलंकार	rgyan	ornament
अल्प	(1) ñuṅ (ba)	a little
	(2) chuṅ	
	(3) cuṅ zad	
अल्पाधिक	bag che	more or less
अवगाह	lums	medicated bath
अवज्ञा	brñas pa	to show disrespect
अवरोध	(1) dgag (pa)	to inhibit, to obstruct
	(2) gnag (pa)	
अशुभ	sdig (pa)	inauspicious
अश्रु	mchi ma	tears
अश्लील	khum	vulgar
अश्व	rta	horse
अश्वारोहण	rta rgyug	horse riding
असात्म्य	mi'phrod (pa)	unwholesome
अस्ति	yod (pa)	to exist
अस्थि	rus (pa)	bone
अस्थिरस	rus khu	bone-soup
अहंकार	ṅa rgyal	pride, ego
अहितकर	(1) gnod (pa)	harmful
	(2) mi 'phrod (pa)	unwholesome

आ

आकर्षण	draṅ (ba)	attraction
आकाश	nam mkha'	sky
आक्रान्त	(1) gzir (ba)	to be afflicted, to suffer,
	(2) gyos pa	to be attacked,
	(3) btab	to be afflicted

आख्यान	bsten pa	explanation
आगम	luṅ	instruction, commandment
आगमन	(1) o'ṅ (ba)	to come, to become
	(2) lhags	in the advent of
आचरण	(1) spyad	to perform
	(2) gyur pa	to become, conduct
आचार्य	(1) ā rya	preceptor
	(2) slob dpon	
आत्मन्	(1) ñid	self
	(2) bdag	
	(3) raṅ	
आत्मभय	raṅ ñam	fear complex
आदान	mar 'bri(b) pa	degeneration
अदानकाल	mar 'bri dus	time of absorption
आदि	la sogs (pa)	etcetera, and others
आदेश	luṅ	instructions
आन्ध्य	mdoṅs (pa)	blindness
आभरण	rgyan	ornament
आमलकी	skyu ru ra	emblic myrobaloon, *Emblica officinalis*
आमाशय	pho ba	stomach
आयास	ṅal ba	fatigue
आयुस्	(1) 'cho (ba)	life
	(2) tshe	
आरोह	srid	hight
आर्द्र	(1) rlon (pa)	wet, green
	(2) rlan	humid, moist
आर्द्रक	sga	ginger, dryginger
आर्य	'phags pa	noble
आवरण	dgab pa	to cover
आवास	gnas	house
आसन	stan	seat
आस्तरण	star gdiṅ	carpet

इ

इति	źes	thus ends.

उ

उत्क्लेशन	draṅ (ba)	to draw out
उत्तम	(1) mchog	the best, excellent
	(2) bsod (pa)	the most agreeable
उत्तमशाक	ldum mchog	the best among vegetables
उत्तिष्ठन	laṅs	to get up
(उत्थित)	(laṅ ba)	
उत्थान	(1) ldaṅ (ba)	to get aggravated, to arise
(उत्पन्न)	(2) 'greṅ (ba)	to stand
उत्पन्न	(1) 'byuṅ (ba)	to give rise to
	(2) 'gyur (ba)	to cause
	(3) sloṅ	to give rise to
उत्पादन	(1) skye ba	producer, aggravator
	(2) bskyed	
उत्साह	'grus pa	enthusiasm
उदर	lto (ba)	abdomen
उदरकृमि	lto'i srin bu	worms in the abdomen
उदरपूर्ण	'graṅs pa	bellyful
उद्घाटन	bsal	release
उद्देश्य	don	object
उद्भव	'byuṅ (ba)	to give rise to
उद्यम	nan tan	professional duty
उपदेश	bstan pa	advice
उपभोग	(1) bsten	to enjoy, to attend
	(2) spyad	
उपरान्त	phyin chad	afterwards
उपवेशन	'dug (pa)	to sit
उपयुक्त	gar mthun	suitable

उष्ण	(1) tsha (ba)	hot, heating
	(2) bsro (ba)	
	(3) tshan mo	
	(4) dron po	
	(5) dro (ba)	
उष्णगृह	bsro khaṅ	warm house, heated house
उष्णजल	chu tsha(n)	hot water
उष्णभोजन	zan dron	warm food
उष्णरस	khu tshan	hot soup
उष्णोदक	chu (dro) 'jam	warm water, tepid water

ऊ

ऊष्मा	drod	heat, digestive stimulant

ऋ

ऋतु	dus	season
ऋषि	draṅ sroṅ	sage, saint

ए

एक	cig (gcig)	one
एकत्र	lhan cig	together
एते	'di rnams	these

ओ

ओष	mos (pa)	dew drops
ओष्ठ	mchu	lip

औ

औषध	sman	medicine
औषधि श्रेष्ठ	sman mchog	the best among medicines

क

कटु	cha (ba)	pungent
कण्डू	(1) gyan pa	itching
	(2) gya' (ba)	
कथन	(1) gsuṅs	speech
	(2) śed	
	(3) smros	
	(4) brjod pa	description
कथा	ṅag	speech, advice
कदा	res 'ga'	at times
कदा कदा	(1) bar bar	at times
	(2) sabs skabs	
कफ	bad kan	*kapha*, one of the three factors controlling body physiology
कम्पन	sprugs	shaking
करका	ser bu	hailstone
करण	bya	to make, to do
कर्कोटी	ga gon	cucumber
कर्ण	rna (ba)	ear
कर्तन	(1) bregs (pa)	to cut
	(2) bcad (pa)	
कर्त्तव्य	(1) bya	duty, to do
	(2) sla	
कर्त्तव्यकर्म	brtsal ba	duty
कर्तित	tog	harvested
कर्म	(1) brtson pa	effort
	(2) las	
कल्याण	dge (ba)	auspicious
कल्याणमित्र	dge bśes (pa)	auspicious friend
कषाय	bskol (ba)	decoction, boiled
कषाय (रस)	bska (ba)	astringent taste
काम	(1) loṅs spyod	passion, sexdesire
	(2) sdod	
	(3) 'dod (pa)	

कारक	(1) ldaṅ (ba)	producer
	(2) bskyed	
	(3) byed (pa)	to produce, to perform
काल (अधिक)	(1) riṅ	(long) time
	(2) dus	time
काष्ठ	śiṅ	wood, twig,
कास	lud pa	caughing
किरण	o'd zer	ray
कुक्कुट	bya	fowl
कुण्ड	khuṅ	pit, cavity
कुमार	sras	son
कृत	byas pa	done, composed
कृमि	srin bu	worm
कृश	skems (pa)	thin, emaciated
कृष्ण	nag po	black
कृष्णधान्य	rgya sran nag po	black-gram
कृष्णपशु	gnag pa	yak, black-cattle
क्रन्दन	ṅud mo	crying
क्रमशः	rim bźin	consecutively, successively
क्रीडा	rtse (ba)	play
क्रूर	drag po	fierceful
क्रोध	(1) khro (ba)	anger
	(2) gtum (po)	
क्लान्त	dub (pa)	fatigue
क्लेश	ñon moṅs (pa)	misery
क्वाथ	bskol (ba)	decoction
क्षवथु	sbrid pa	sneezing
क्षुधा	bkres (pa)	hunger

ख

खण्ड	kha ṇḍa	solid extact in the form of paste.
खण्डित	ban bun	broken
खरस्रोतस्	bzad po	having strong current

ग

गत	thag	to become,to pass over
गन्ध	dri	smell
गमन	'gro (ba)	to go, walk
गुड	bu ram	jaggery
गुडूची	sle tres	*Tinospora cordifolia*
गुफा	phug pa	cave
गुरु	(1) lci (ba)	heavy
	(2) rje dpon	preceptor
गुल्म	skran	phantom tumour
गोक्षुर	gze ma	*Tribulus terrestris*
गोधूम	gro	wheat
गृंजनक	ke'u	carrot
गृह	(1) gnas	house
	(2) khaṅ (ba)	
	(3) khyim	domesticated
गृहकुक्कुट	khyim bya	domesticated fowl
ग्रहण	bab	to take
ग्रीवा	mdziṅ	neck
ग्रीष्म	dbyar	summer
ग्रीष्मपूर्वभाग	dbyar stod	first part of summer
ग्रीष्मोत्तरभाग	dbyar smad	later part of summer

घ

घर्षण	brud	rubbing
घृणा	spyi brtol	hatred
घृत	(1) źun mar	ghee, melted butter
	(2) mar khu	

च

चक्षु	mig	eye
चण्ड	gñan pa	fierceful
चतुष्पथ	lam mdo	cross-road
चत्वार	bźi	four
चन्द्र	zla ba	moon

चन्द्रग्रहण	(?) zla ba spyaṅ kyis zin	lunar eclipse
चर्म्मरी	gnag pa	yak
चर्या	(1) tshul	conduct
	(2) spyod tshul	
	(3) spyod (lam)	
चित्त	sems	mind
चिन्तन	bsam (pa)	to think
चिह्न	rtags	sign
चैत्य	mchod rtan	religious monument of Buddhists
चंक्रमण	bcag	walking

छ

छत्रक	śa mo	mushroom
छन्द	tshigs	metrices, verse
छाया	grib ma	shadow

ज

जनक	(1) skye (ba)	producer
	(2) skyed (pa)	aggravator
जनन	(1) 'gyur (ba)	to produce, to cause
	(2) skyes pa	
जरा	rgas (pa)	old age, aging process
जल	chu	water
जलकुक्कुट	chu bya	water fowl
जलमिश्रिततक्र	dar chus bslad	butter-milk mixed with water
जांगलदेश	skam sa	arid land, dry land
जात	skyes	birth
जीर्ण	źu (ba)	digestion
जीर्णमूलक	la phug rñiṅ	over matured radish
जीवन	'tsho ba	life
जीवसूत्र	Dzi ba sūtra	n. of this work, lit. principle of healthy living
जूर्णाह्व	tsi	millet

जृम्भा	(1) g'yal	yawning
	(2) glal (ba)	
ज्ञान	(1) śes pa	to know
	(2) rig pa	knowledge
	(3) rtogs (pa)	known
ज्येष्ठ	dbyar	n. of a month (April-May)
ज्येष्ठमास	dbyar zla	
ज्वर	rims	fever

झ

झर	chu mig	spring

त

तक्र	dar (ra)	butter-milk
तत्	de	that
तत्काल	de riṅ	at that time
तथा	(1) de ltaṅ	like that
	(de ltar yaṅ)	
	(2) de ltar	
तद्	'di	that
तदनन्तर	(1) de las	thereafter
	(2) de nas	
	(3) de rjes	
तदर्थ	de phyir	for that
तप्त	gtuṅ (ba)	to be scortched
तरुण	ma laṅs	immature
तर्क	rtog (pa)	argument
तल	mthil	bottom, sale (of foot).
तिक्त	kha (ba)	bitter
तिब्बती भाषा	Bod skad	Tibetan language
तिल	ti la	sessame
तीक्ष्ण	(1) rno (ba)	sharp
	(2) phra sṅags	
	(3) drag po	

तीव्र	myos pa	strong, intoxicating
तुषार	(1) zil pa	dew, frost
	(2)mos pa	
तैल	mar	oil
त्याग	(1) 'dzem	to avoid
	(2) dor (ba)	to throw out
	(3) spaṅ(s) (ba)	to give up
त्रय	gsum	three

द

दग्ध	bsregs (pa)	burnt
दधि	źo	curd
दन्त	so	tooth
दन्तकाष्ठ	so śiṅ	twig for brushing teeth
दन्तविद्रधि	so na śu ba	gum abscess, tumour in tooth
दर्शन	(1) lta (ba)	to look at
	(2) blta	
दश	bcu	ten
दशमंगलकर्म	dge bcu	ten auspicious efforts
दाडिम	bal po se'u	pomegranate
दारण	bri ('bri ba)	to scratch, to draw
दारुहरिद्रा	skyer pa	*Berberis aristata*
दार्वीरसांजन	skyer pa'i kha ṇḍa	solid extract from *Berberis aristata*
दिवा	(1) ñi ma	day-time
	(2) ñin (mo)	
	(3) ñin (pa)	
दिवानिन्द्रा	ñin par log	day-sleep
दीपन	drod	digestive stimulant
दीर्घायुस्	tshe riṅ	longevity
दुःख	mya ṅan	sorrow
दुग्ध	o' (ma)	milk
दूषण	gnod pa	vitiation
दृष्ट	brtsam pa	found
देव	lha	God

देश	(1) yul	place of habitation
	(2) rgya	country
दोष	(1) ñes pa	morbid factors in the body
	(2) skyon	fault, defect
द्राक्षा	rgun ('brum)	grape
द्राक्षासव	rgun chaṅ	alocholic preparation of grapes.
द्वय	gñis	two
द्वेष	dpyas (pa)	to find fault with others

ध

धर्म	chos	religion
धान्य	'bru	corn, cereals
धारण	(1) byug pa	to wear
	(2) gdags	to carry
धावन	baṅ	running
धी	blo	wisdom
धूम	dud pa	smoke
धूलि	rdul	dust
ध्वज	rgyal mtshan	flag

न

न	(1) mi	no, negative indicator
	(2)min	
	(3)ma	
नख	sen mo	nails
नदीजल	chu grog	river-water
नदीतट	grog	river bank, ravine
नमस्	phyag 'tshal (ba)	to bow before
नम्र	sma	humble, polite
नव	gsar tog	freshly harvested
नवनीत	mar (g)sar	fresh butter
नागार्जुन	Klu-sgrub	n. of a Buddhist saint and expounder of Mādhyamika philosophy

नागार्जुनहृदय	Klu-sgrub-sñin-po	n. of a Buddhist saint
निकट	druṅ	near
निखिल	kun	all
निगदित	brjod (pa)	stated
निद्रा	(1) ñal (ba)	sleep
	(2) log	
	(3) gñid kyis log	
	(4) ñal po	
	(5) gñid	
निन्द्य	ldam ldum	not useful
निमित्त	ched	because of
नियमन	(1) srid	govern
	(2) dbaṅ bsgyur (ba)	
निराकरण	sel (ba)	to remove, to cleanse, to cure
निर्मल	(1) gtsaṅ (ba)	free from impurity.
	(2) dri ma med	clean
निर्लज्ज	spyi brtol	shameless
निर्विष	dug med	free from poison
निर्हरण	(1) dbyuṅ pa	to take out
	(2) sel (ba)	to remove, to clear
निवात	bser bu mi phog	free from wind
निवास	(1) 'dug (pa)	to reside
	(2) bca' (ba)	
निश्चय	ṅes (pa)	to ensure
नीच	dman	mean
नीली	ram ñe	indigo

प

पक्व	laṅs (laṅ ba)	matured
पक्षी	bya	bird
पंचत्रिंशत्	sum cu rtsa lṅa	thirty five
पंचपंचाशत्	lṅa bcu lṅa	fifty five
पठन	(1) yi ge klog	to study
	(2)klog pa	

थ	lam	road
द्य	tshigs	verse
रस्पर	phan tshun	each other
रिधान	(1) byas pa (2)gdags (3)bgo (ba)	to wear
रिधि	sgor	compound
रिवार	'khor	retinue, family
रिहास	dgod (pa)	jest, joke
रीक्षा	(1) brtag (pa) (2)dpyad (dpyod pa)	to examine
रुष	rtsub (pa)	coarse
र्वत	ri	mountain
लाण्डु	btsoṅ	onion
वित्र	gtsaṅ (ba)	free from impurity
श्चात्	(1) naṅ nub (2)nub	afterwards
श्चात्ताप	chad (pa)	repentance
श्चाद्भाग	smad	later part
क	'ju (ba)	digestion
द	rkaṅ (pa)	foot
प	sdig (pa)	sin
न	(1) 'thuṅ(s) (2)gnon (pa) (3)btuṅ (ba)	to drink
लन	bruṅ (ba)	to follow
षाण	rdo	stone
ता	pha	father
त्त	mkhris pa	one of the three morbidity causing factors in the body
पासा	skom	thirst
त	ser (ka)	yellow
तभाग	spri	yalk or yellow portion of the egg
डन	brdab (pa)	to press, to squeeze

पीड़ा	gnod (pa)	pain
पुनः	skyor (ba)	again
पुराण	(1) rñiṅ (pa)	old, over matured
	(2) lha (ba)	stale, preserved for a long time
पुराणगुड	bu ram rñid	old jaggery
पुराणघृत	mar rñiṅ	old ghee
पुराणमद्य	chaṅ rñiṅ	old wine
पुराणसर्षप	yuṅs rñiṅ	old mustard
पुरीष	bśaṅ (ba)	stool
पुरुष	skyes bu	man, human being
पुष्कर	ma nu	Inula racemosa
पुष्करबीज	ma nu'i sa bon	seed of *Inula racemosa*
पूजन	(1) mchod (pa) (2)khyud (pa)	prayer, worship
पूज्य	sri źu (ba)	respect
पूति	lha (ba)	stale, putrified, preserved for a long time
पूरण	blugs	to pour
पूर्व	(1) stod	first part
	(2) sṅar	before
पूर्वकृत	sṅar bya	efforts of the past
पूर्वभाग	'sar (ba)	early part
पूर्वाभिभाषी	gsoṅ (po,	to wish others before one is wished
पेशल	des (pa)	noble conduct
प्रकृति	rtags	characteristic features, signs and symptoms
प्रकोप	ldaṅ (ba)	to get aggravated
प्रक्षालन	(1) bśal (ba) (2)bkru	to wash
प्रज्ञा	blo	wisdom, intellect
प्रणिपात	(1) gtod (pa) (2)phyag 'tshal (ba)	to surrender
प्रतिश्याय	cham pa	cold, influenza
प्रतिस्पर्धा	'gran (pa)	competition

त्यूष	(1) tho rans	dawn
	(2)skya reṅ	
	(3)dmar thag	
त्यूषप्रथमभाग	skya reṅs śar (ba)	early part of dawn
थम	gcig pa	first
थम भाग	śar (ba)	early part
दर्शन	(1) bstan	exhibit
	(2)bcag	
	(3)bstan	
देश	ñi che	place of habitation.
भृति	la sogs (pa)	etcetera, and others
यत्न	brtson pa	to strive
योग	(1) btaṅ	administration
	(2)gtaṅ (ba)	
वचन	gtam	religious speeches
वेश	(1) loṅ (pa)	to arrive at
	(2) dbab (pa)	to enter into
शम	(1) bsal	allevriation, cure
	(2)sel (ba)	
ांजलि आसन	tsog bu (pu)	squatting with folded hands
ाण	sems	life
ाणी	(1) phyugs	animal
	(2)sems can	
	(3)srog chags	
ाणीवसा	phyags mar	animal fat
ातः	naṅ par	morning
ाप्त	thob pa	to obtain
ाप्ति	'gyur (ba)	to acquire
ार्थना	mchod (pa)	prayer
ावृट्ट	dbyar smad	later part of summer
ेरण	bskrus	to incite

फ

फल	śiṅ tog	fruit
फाफर	bra po	buck-wheat

ब

बलि	gtor ma	sacrificial offering
बहिस्	phyi	outside
बहु	maṅ (po) (ba)	more, much
बारम्बार	s'kabs skabs	frequently
बालक	byis pa	child
बिन्दु (?)	zer ma	drop
बीज	sa bon	seed
बुद्धि	blo	intellect
बृहत्	chen po	big
बृहत् पाषाण	pha boṅ	big boulder

भ

भक्षण	(1) 'gam (pa)	eating
	(2) zos (za ba)	to eat
	(3) bca' (ba)	to chew (for brushing)
भंग	(1) gźom (pa)	to break
	(2)bcag	
भद्र	(1) des (pa)	gentle, noble
	(2) su	auspicious
भय	ñam	fear
भर्जित	(1) bsreg (pa)	fried
	(2)brdos (pa)	
भस्म	thal (ba)	ashes.
भस्मकुण्ड	thal khuṅ	place of or cavity for ashes
भाग	(1) bam po	section, group of chapters
	(2) cha	part
भाण्ड	snod	vessel
भारत	Rgya-gar	India
भारतीयभाषा	Rgya-gar skad	Indian language, Sanskrit
भावना	dgoṅs pa	thought
भाषण	smra ba	speech
भाषा	skad	language
भिक्षु	dge sloṅ	monk

भिषक्	sman pa	physician
भिषक् श्रेष्ठ	sman pa'i mchog	best among the physicians
भूमि	sa	land
भृष्टयव	yos	roasted barley
भैषज्य	sman	medicine
भोग	loṅs spyod	enjoyment
भोजन	(1) dro (2)zan (3)bag (4)bza' (ba) (5)zas	meal
भोजनग्रहण	dro bab	to take food
भोटभाषा	Bod - skad	Tibetan language

म

मंगल	gyuṅ (druṅ)	auspicious, benedictory
मणि	rin chen	gems and jewels
मण्डल	ma ṇḍa la	mystic and sacred circle
मति	blo	mind
मतिमान्	blo ldan pa	wise man
मत्त	(1) myos pa (2)ra ro	intoxicated
मत्स्य	ña	fish
मद्य	chaṅ	alcoholic drink
मधु	sbraṅ rtsi	honey
मधुर	mnar (ba)	sweet
मधूदक	sbra chu	water mixed with honey
मध्य	bar	intermediate period
मध्यम	'briṅ po	mediocre, middle
मध्याह्ण	ñi ma phyed	midday
मध्वासव	sbraṅ chaṅ	alcoholic drink prepared of honey
मनस्	(1) yid (2)sems	mind
मनोरम	yid du o'ṅ	friendly
मन्त्र	sṅags	sacred incantation

मन्द	dub (pa)	mild
मन्दिर	lha khaṅ	temple
मरिच	na le śam	black pepper, piper nigrum
मल	(1) slo	stool
	(2) dri ma	dirt
महत्	che (ba)	much in excess
महर्षि	draṅ sroṅ chen po	great sage
महान्	chen po	great
महावृक्ष	śiṅ chen	big tree
मांस	śa	meat
माता	(1) ma	mother
	(2)yum	
मान	tsad	span, measurement
मानव	mi	man
माया	sgyu ma	illusion
मार्ग	lam	road
मार्जन	byi dor	cleansing
माष	rgya sran nag po	black-gram
मित	ran (pa)	appropriately
मित्र	(1) bśes pa	friend
	(2)sri żu (ba)	
	(3)grogs	
मिश्रण	(1) 'dre (ba)	to mix
	(2) 'phrad (pa)	mixture
	(3) bsre (ba)	
	(4) bslad (pa)	
	(5) 'dres pa	
	(6) btab	to add
	(7) blugs	to pour
मुख	(1) gdoṅ	face
	(2) kha	mouth
मुद्ग	mu ka	*Phaseolus mungo*
मुनि	brtul żugs (can)	an ascetic
मूत्र	gci (ba)	urine
मूलक	la phug	radish
मृग	śa pa	large stag

मृतदेह	ro	dead body
मृत्यु	'chi ba	death
मृदु	'jam	soft
मेदस्	tsil	fat
मेदस्वी	tson	fatty
मेष	lug	sheep
मेषवसा	lug gi mar	sheep-fat
मैत्री	byams pa	friendship
मैथुन	ñal po	sexual intercourse
मोक्षण	dbyuṅ pa	to take out
मोह	gi mug	illusion

य

यकृत्	mchin pa	liver
यत् किंचित्	gaṅ yaṅ	whatsoever
यत्र	yin yaṅ	wherever
यथा	(1) bźin	according as
	(2) ci	what
	(3) ji ltar	in whatsoever manner
यथायोग्य	(1) ci raṅ	appropriately
	(2) raṅ (pa)	
यथांयोग्य भावना	ñer bsam	appropriate respect
यदा	na	when
यदि	yaṅ	if
यव	nas	barley
यवागू	skyo ma	thin gruel
यश	grags	fame
युक्त	(1) can	suffix meaning possessed with
	(2) btab	added with
	(3) yod pa	to exist
यूष	thug pa	vegetable soup
यौवन	(1) dar	youth
	(2) laṅ tshe	

र

रक्त	dmar (po)	red colour
रक्तमोक्षण	khrag dbyuṅ pa	blood-letting
रक्षण	bsruṅ (ba)	to protect
रचित	bcad (pa)	composed
रमण	rgyo	indulgence in sex
रस	(1) ro	taste
	(2) khu ba	soup
	(3) bro (ba)	taste
रसयुक्त	ro yod	delicious
रसांजन	staṅ zil	antimony
रहित	(1) mi ldaṅ	free from
	(2) med (pa)	without
राजनियम	bka' khrims	commandment, kings orders
राजा	rgyal po	king
रात्रि	(1) nam	night
	(2) nam sros	
रुक्ष	rtsub (pa)	rough, coarse
रुद्र	drag po	fierceful
रोगी	nad can	patient
रोध	mnan	to subdue, obstruction

ल

लक्षण	rtags	sign
लघु	yaṅ (ba) (po)	light
लवण	(1) lan tshwa	salt
	(2) tsa (tshwa)	
लशुन	sgog skya	garlic
लिंग	rtags	sign
लेप	bsku	rubbing, application

व

वक	bya gag	crane
वचा	śu dag	*Acorus calamus*

वध	bsad pa	killing
वन्यमरिच	g'yer (ma)	wild capsicum
वन्यमुद्ग	ka tsam	wild oat
वमन	skyug (pa)	emesis
वमनकर्म	skyug sman	emetic therapy
वराह	phag pa	boar
वर्णन	'dom	description
वर्ष	lo	year
वर्षा	char pa	rain
वसन्त	dpyid	spring
वसा	tshil	fat
वस्त्र	gos	cloth
वहन	gdags	to carry
वाक् (वाणी)	(1) tsig (2) ṅag	talk, speech
वात	(1) bser bu (2) ṅad	wind
वातल	ṅad can	windy
वात्या	drag po'i ṅad	strong wind
वायु	rluṅ	one of the three morbid factors in the body
वार्धक्य	rgas	aging process, old age
वाहय	phyi rol	outside
विंशति	ñi śu	twenty
विकारि	sgyu ma	perversion
विद्या	rigs pa	knowledge
विद्रधि	śu ba	abscess
विना	min	except, without
विपरीत	(1) med pa (2) log	opposite (2)
विपरीत भाषण	med smra (ba)	negative speaking
विरेचन	bkru	purgation
विरचनकर्म	bkru sman	purgation therapy
विविध	sna tshogs	different types
विशेषतया	khyed pa	specially, particularly
विश्राम	'dug (pa)	to take rest

विष	dug	poison
विस्तार	(1) snar	expansion
	(2) brta (ba)	to expand
विस्फोटक	śu ba	blister
विहार	(1) bźugs	to exist
	(2) bag	regimens
वृक्ष	śiṅ	tree
वृद्ध	(1) rgan (po)	old
	(2) rñiṅ (pa)	over matured
वृद्धा	bud med rgan	old woman
वेदी	stegs	seat of the gods and saints
वैद्यजीवसूत्र	Sman 'tsho ba'i mdo	n. of this work
व्यतिरिक्त	ma gtogs (pa)	with the exception of
व्यवाय	ñal po	sexual intercourse
व्याधि	nad	disease
व्यायाम	(1) bskyod (pa)	exercise
	(2) ṅal ba	
व्रतिन्	brtul źugs (can)	sage

श

शक्ति	nus pa	strength
शक्तु	(1) phye	roasted corn-flour
	(2) zan dron	
शब्द	smra ba	noise
शयन	ñal po	sleep
शरत्	ston	autumn
शरीर	lus	body
शर्करा	kha ra (ka ra)	sugar
शव	(1) dur (ba)	dead body
	(2) mi ro	
शशक	ri boṅ	rabbit
शाक	ldum	vegetables
शान्ति	zi ba	to get alleviated, to be pacified

शालि	'bras	rice
शासन	(1) bka'	instruction
	(2) bstan pa	explanation
शिक्षा	bslab	education
शिखर	sna	top
शिम्बीधान्य	sran ma	pulse
शिरस्	mgo (bo)	head
शिराव्यध	gtar ka (ga)	venesection
शिशिर	dgun smad	later part of winter
शिशु	byis pa	child
शीघ्र	(1) mgyos (pa)	quickly
	(2) bab chol	
	(3) myur (ba)	
शीत	(1) bsil (ba)	cold, cooling
	(2) gsil (ba)	
	(3) graṅ (ba)	
शीतकाल	dgun	winter
शीतल	grog	cold
शीतलजल	chu grog	cold water
शीतवात	ser bu	cold wind
शीर्ण	draṅs	emaciation
शील	tshul	conduct
शुक्र	khu chu	semen
शुक्ल	dkar (po)	white, pure
शुचि	gcaṅ (ba)	free from impurity
शुण्ठी	sga	dry ginger
शुण्ठ्युदक	sga chu	water boiled with ginger
शुभदान	gtoṅ (ba)	auspicious charity
शुष्क	skam (pa)	arid, dry
शुष्कमांस	śa skam	dry-meat
शून्यस्थान	stoṅ (pa)	empty space
शृत	bskol (ba)	boiled
शोधन	(1) sbyaṅ ba	cleansing
	(2) bkru	
	(3) byi dor	
	(4) bsal	

श्रम	ṅal ba	fatigue
श्मशान	dur khrod	cemetery
श्रमण	dge (ba) sbyoṅ	religious ascetic
श्रवण	(1) mñan (pa)	to hear
	(2) sñan	
	(3) thos (pa)	
श्रेष्ठ	mchog	the best, the excellent
श्वास	dbugs mi bde	dyspnoea, asthma

ष

षट्	drug	six

स

संकोचन	gcu (ba)	contraction, squeezing
संक्रमण	ldaṅ (ba)	to spread
संक्रामक रोग	rims	infectious disease, fever
संक्षेप	(1) bag byed	brief
	(2) mdor	
संगीत	sgra	music
संचय	gsog (pa)	accumulation
सत्त्व	sems	spirit
सदा	cir	always
सद्य	ma thag	immediately after maturity
सन्निहित	bźugs	to remain
सन्तोष	noms pa	satisfaction
सन्ध्या	(1) sros	evening
	(2) chad (pa)	dusk
सन्यास	chad (pa)	to be free from worldly bondage
सभक्ति श्रवण	sñan mñan	to hear with devotion
सम	(1) raṅ (pa)	appropriately
	(2) mñam	equally
समभाग	cha mñam	equal part
समय	(1) tshe	time, life
	(2) dus	

समाप्ति	rdzogs	completion
समासतः	mdor	in brief.
सामुद्रलवण	rgyam tsha	sea salt
सम्पर्क	phog	to come in contact
सम्मान	(1) sri (2) sri źu (ba)	respect
सम्यक्	ran (pa)	appropriately
सर्प	sbrul	snake
सर्व	kun	all
सर्वज्ञ	Thams cad mkhyen pa	Omniscient
सर्षप	yuṅs	mustard
सर्षपतैल	yuṅs mar	mustard oil
सशक्त	drag tu	violently
संस्कृतभाषा	Rgya-gar-skad	Sanskrit language
सह	(1) bcas (2) lhan	together with
सात्म्य	'phrod (pa)	wholesome
साधन	(1) sbub pa (2) bsgrub	performance, practice
सामान्यकर्म	rtsol bcag	normal efforts, work
सात्म्योत्पादक	sñoms	to bring harmony
सांय	(1) srod (2) nub mo	dusk, evening
सारत्व	sra (ba)	compactness
साहस	(1) rtsal (2) stobs	exhibition of strength
सिक्त	gśer ba	to get drenched
सिंघाणक	snabs	nasal excretion
सिद्ध	ya mtshan	mystic
सुकर	sla	easy to perform
सुख	(1) bde (ba) (2) dgar (dga' bar) (3) so (4) skyid (pa)	happiness, contentment

सुखोदक	chu dro	luke-warm water
सुखोष्ण	ran dro	luke-warm
सुगन्ध	dri źim (pa)	agreeable smell
सुन्दर	mdzes (pa)	beautiful
सुपाच्य	'ju sla (ba)	easily digestible
सुरामण्ड	caṅ chu	upper portion of alcoholic drink
सूत्र	mdo	rule, axiom, statement in brief
सूर्य	ñi ma	sun
सेव	ku su	apple
सेवन	(1) spyad	to resort to
	(2) gtaṅ (ba)	
	(3) bsten	to attend
सौन्दर्य (?)	rma	beauty
स्त्री	(1) bag (ma)	wife
	(2) bu med	woman
स्थान	(1) yul	place of habitation
	(2) sa	land
	(3) gnas	house
स्थित	bźag (pa)	to exist, to remain
स्थूल	gźag (pa) stug	thick
स्नान	(1) bkru	bath
स्निग्ध (स्नेह)	(2) mar	unctuous, oily
	snum pa	
स्निग्धभोजन	snum bag	unctuous food
स्नेह	chags (pa)	love, attachment
स्पर्श	reg (pa)	touch, to expose
स्फुटिका	lce myaṅ tsha	alum
स्मित	'dzum	smiling
स्वयं	(1) raṅ	self
	(2) 'dra	
स्वस्तिक	g'yuṅ (druṅ)	auspicious, benedictory
स्वेदन	dugs	fomentation

ह

हरिण	rgya	deer
हरीतकी	a ru ra	*Terminalia chebula*
हस्त	lag pa	hand
हास्य	(1) gad mo	laughter
	(2) ya mtshan	to ridicule
हिक्का	skigs pa	hiccup
हित	phan pa	benefit
हितकर	'phrod (pa)	useful
हीन	dman	mean
हृदय	sñiṅ (po)	heart
हेमन्त	dgun stod	first part of winter
हेतु	phyir	reason, because of
होमकुण्ड	ho ma khuṅ	place for sacrificial offerings
ह्रद	mtsho	lake